Mental Wellness
The Secret Ingredients

Mental Wellness
The Secret Ingredients

A 10-Step Holistic Guide
Grounded in Science

By
Colby J. C. Bryce

Registered Psychologist
Registered Nutritionist
Researcher & Scientist

ISBN: 978-1-7637544-0-9 (paperback)
ISBN: 978-1-7637544-2-3 (Kindle)

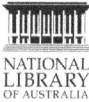 A catalogue record for this book is available from the National Library of Australia

NATIONAL LIBRARY OF AUSTRALIA

Printed and bound in Australia, United States or United Kingdom by IngramSpark, Lightning Source Inc.

Cover design and Illustrations: Kylie Dunn, kyliedunn.com

Edited by: Merridy Pugh, Dr Liz Charpleix, Amara Motala

Contents

This book is dedicated to those who are navigating their way through their own unique mental health challenges. Your resilience and courage inspire me to continue striving for understanding, empathy, and progress in the field of mental health.

If you've ever felt isolated in your experience, I hope this guide offers support, compassion, and practical advice. Your path is unique, and your challenges are valid. Remember, seeking help and working towards better mental health is a brave step, and every effort you make brings you closer to your own version of wellbeing.

To the families and friends supporting loved ones experiencing mental health difficulties: your care is incredibly important. This guide is also for you—to acknowledge your impact and help you better understand and assist those you care about.

To the professionals dedicated to helping others, your work is invaluable. I hope this guide adds to the collective effort to enhance understanding and support for those in need.

Together, with empathy and unity, we can make a difference in the lives of those facing mental health challenges.

Introduction

"Mental health is not a destination, but a process. It's about how you drive, not where you're going." Noam Shpancer, Doctor of Clinical Psychology

Think of this guide as your driving instructor, but instead of helping you navigate the road, it's here to help you navigate your mental health. It's packed with tips and strategies, but ultimately, it's up to you to take control and apply what you learn.

Learning to support your mental health is one of the most valuable things you can do. Starting this process might be tough, but it's definitely worth it. Remember, there's no final destination where you just stop working on your mental health. It's an ongoing process, and you'll need to keep using the strategies in this guide to stay on track.

Being open to change is key. As Charles Darwin wisely said, *"It's not the strongest or the smartest that survive, but those who adapt best to change."* This idea applies to mental health too—those who embrace change often find more contentment. Persistence is also important. Research suggests that habits typically take about 60 days to develop or break, so be patient with yourself and accept that setbacks are part of the process.

Historically, Western medicine has focused on symptoms and illnesses, while traditional psychology often zeroes in on disorders rather than overall wellbeing. This guide seeks to shift that perspective by providing a program designed to help you achieve and maintain optimal mental health, rather than just addressing symptoms.

Many mental health guides and self-help books dive deep into complex strategies or focus too narrowly on one aspect of wellbeing. If you're struggling, you might not have the energy to sift through a dozen books. That's why this guide offers a simple, all-in-one, holistic approach. It breaks things down into manageable steps, presenting them in a logical order to make it easier for you to support your mental health effectively.

Through this holistic approach, I'll be here to support you as a whole person, looking at your emotional, physical, social, cognitive, and spiritual wellbeing. I use different methods and support systems that focus on the areas most affecting your mental health, rather than just zeroing in on specific symptoms or disorders.

I've designed the guide to help you take things one step at a time, with each part building on the previous one. By following the steps in order, you'll find it easier to support your mental health.

While developing this guide, I drew on the latest research and I have applied this to clients, friends, family, and even my own experience to create this roadmap, so you can navigate the path to better mental wellbeing.

Congratulations on starting your journey towards your ideal version of mental health today—think of it as the start of your road trip!

How will this guide help with my mental wellness?

Think of working with this guide as being like cooking your favourite meal. Each step is like an ingredient or instruction in the recipe. Some steps are more crucial than others, but each one adds something essential to the final dish. This guide provides you with a recipe for optimal mental health.

Here's the 10-step recipe for wellness:

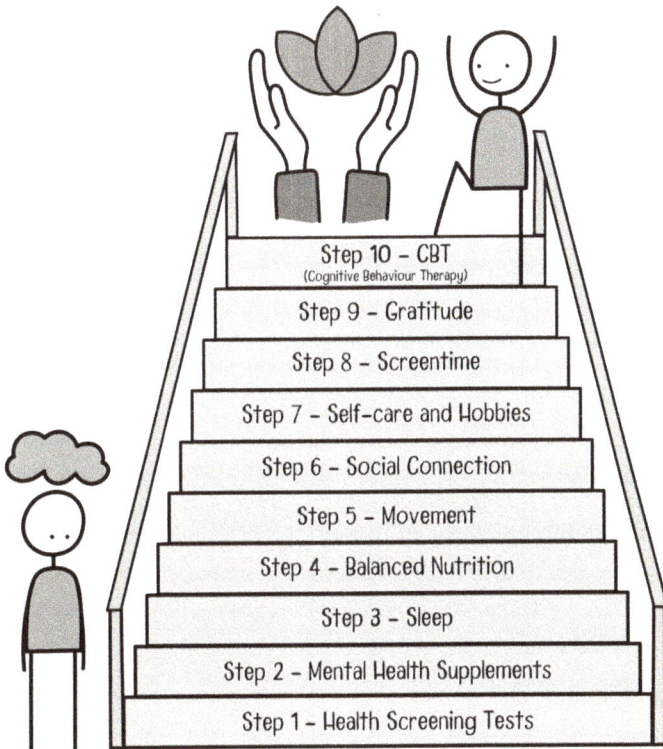

Step 10 – CBT
(Cognitive Behaviour Therapy)

Step 9 – Gratitude

Step 8 – Screentime

Step 7 – Self-care and Hobbies

Step 6 – Social Connection

Step 5 – Movement

Step 4 – Balanced Nutrition

Step 3 – Sleep

Step 2 – Mental Health Supplements

Step 1 – Health Screening Tests

1. Check out recommended mental health-based screening tests including vitamin D.
2. Review supplements that are known to support mental health.
3. Learn how to improve your sleep.
4. Maximise your mental health nutrition.
5. Explore the benefits of movement.
6. Understand the importance of social connections.
7. Dive into self-care and hobbies.
8. Discover ways to cut down on screen time.
9. Explore the benefits of gratitude.
10. Use cognitive behaviour therapy in the comfort of your own home.

This guide is designed to help you identify symptoms, uncover potential causes, and change personal behaviours to boost your mental wellness. Each of the 10 steps ends with a list of practical strategies to enhance that step.

After completing the main 10 steps, you'll find additional complementary approaches—think of these as the salt and pepper—to further benefit your mental health.

You can work through each step at your own pace. The guide breaks down each step into smaller, more manageable tasks and presents them in a logical order, making it easy for you to follow.

By integrating the tasks and insights from each step into your daily life, you'll have a chance to improve your mental health holistically. These steps cover a wide range of techniques to address different aspects of your life, promoting long-term and sustainable wellbeing.

What's the research and science behind this guide?

Each step in this guide is grounded in robust scientific research, primarily from meta-analyses and systematic reviews. These study types pull together results from many individual studies to give you the most reliable and comprehensive conclusions on each topic. The research overview section of this book also includes brief summaries of each reference for those interested in more specific study details. I've included the full names of the lead authors of each study both within the text and as headers for each reference in the research section, making it easier for you to match the research discussed with detailed study information.

What qualifies me to write this guide?

I'm deeply passionate about psychology, which led me to earn 3 degrees in the field: a Bachelor of Psychological Science, a Graduate Diploma of Psychology, and a Master of Applied Psychology. I also hold a bachelor's degree in nutrition, health promotion, and physical activity and health, having spent a total of 8 years at university exploring these areas.

Professionally, I've worked in various mental health settings, from an elite national sports team and clinical psychology practice to centres involved in behaviour analysis and positive behaviour support, a suicide prevention centre, and a research centre at a world-leading university. My work has been published in respected international journals, reflecting my understanding of effective mental health approaches.

Combining my education, professional experiences, and research, I've developed practical strategies for improving mental health. I've seen these methods work in real life with diverse individuals, including clients, friends, family, and myself. Now, it's your turn to benefit from these strategies. With this guide, you're taking an important step towards long-term mental wellbeing. Start reading today and begin your journey to a healthier you.

Understanding Mental Health

To kick things off, let's look at how common mental health challenges really are. According to the World Health Organization, about 1 in 8 people worldwide, which is roughly 970 million individuals, is dealing with a current mental health condition. To put that in perspective, it's around 37 times the entire population of Australia.

There are over 200 different types of mental health disorders, with anxiety and depression being the most prevalent. In fact, about 50% of people with depression also experience anxiety, and vice versa. As of 2019, a staggering 301 million people globally were struggling with anxiety disorders, while 280 million were living with depression. Generalised anxiety disorder is the most common type of anxiety disorder, and major depressive disorder is the most common type of depression.

It's also likely that many more people are dealing with general mental health symptoms that don't quite fit the criteria for a specific diagnosis.

So, if you're finding yourself struggling with mental health, remember: you're definitely not alone. Let's now dive into what might be causing these mental health symptoms.

What influences mental health?

To get a head start on improving mental health and wellbeing, it's important to understand what might be affecting your mental state. You're aiming for a time when you felt happy, calm, and content, but what might be preventing that?

The causes of poor mental health are diverse and unique to everyone, so it's a broad topic. For this guide, I'll give a quick rundown using the biopsychosocial model. This model, introduced by George L. Engel in 1977, was a big and important shift from the old medical model that saw mental illness strictly as a disease. The newer model takes a more holistic view, recognising that our thoughts, feelings, behaviours, history, and genetics all interact in complex ways.

The biopsychosocial model breaks down mental health influences into 3 main areas:

- **Biological:** This includes genetics and brain chemistry.
- **Psychological:** This covers things such as cognition, emotions, personality, and behaviours.
- **Social:** This involves factors such as environmental stressors, socioeconomic status, and social support.

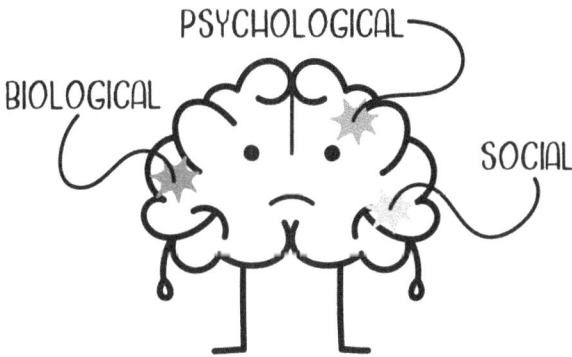

Understanding these factors can help you pinpoint what might be impacting your mental health and guide you towards solutions.

The biopsychosocial model considers the dynamic and interconnected nature of our biology, psychology, and social environment. For example, our biological makeup can influence our thoughts and social interactions, while our thoughts and social experiences can, in turn, affect our biological processes. This model encourages a well-rounded and comprehensive approach to improving mental health. William Lugg from the Royal Prince Alfred Hospital points out that this model is widely used in today's healthcare system. It helps psychologists, psychiatrists, clinicians, researchers, and policymakers understand the complexity of mental health issues and develop interventions that consider the many factors affecting a person's wellbeing.

While the biopsychosocial model provides a helpful framework for understanding the roots of mental health issues, it's important to remember that these challenges often result from a complex interaction of factors. For example, neurotransmitter imbalances might not be the sole cause of mental health conditions, but they can play a significant role in the development and intensity of symptoms. That's why treatment often includes medications to address these imbalances, along with therapy and lifestyle changes to support overall mental health.

It's important to have a basic understanding of the biopsychosocial factors that influence mental health, as the steps within this guide will refer to these elements. Knowing about these factors will help you see why taking those steps can positively impact your mental health. First, we'll break down each component of the biopsychosocial model to give you a clearer picture.

What biological factors impact our mental health?

Biological factors have a significant impact on our mental health, as they're tied to our physical health, genetics, brain chemistry, and hormones. For instance, the genes we inherit can influence how we deal with mental health challenges and how our brains respond to different situations.

Neurotransmitters, the chemicals in our brain, are particularly important in this process. These chemicals are crucial for regulating mood and behaviour, which is why many antidepressants aim to balance them. Here's a closer look at how these common biological factors affect our mental wellbeing.

Neurotransmitters: These are chemicals that transmit signals between nerve cells in our brains, influencing our mood and behaviour. For example, serotonin helps regulate mood and sleep, dopamine is tied to feelings of pleasure and motivation, and norepinephrine is involved in focus and stress management. When these chemicals are balanced, they can support mental wellbeing, but when they are out of balance, they can contribute to mental health issues. That's why medications such as antidepressants are sometimes used to help correct these imbalances. Other important neurotransmitters for mental health include endorphins, which are linked to pain relief and pleasure; oxytocin, which is related to bonding and social interactions; and gamma-aminobutyric acid (GABA), which helps with calming the nervous system.

Inflammation: Inflammation, such as C-reactive protein levels, plays a role in our mental health outcomes. Maintaining balanced inflammation levels keeps our brains in top shape, contributing to our overall mood stability.

Sleep: Sleep quality influences mood, cognitive function, and emotional regulation, potentially impacting stress levels, irritability, and symptoms of anxiety and depression, all of which affect overall mental wellbeing.

Nutrition: The foods we eat play a significant role in our mental health, affecting mood and energy, underscoring the connection between diet and mental health.

Hormones: Hormones, including cortisol, thyroid and sex hormones (e.g. testosterone), play a big part in how we feel by regulating mood, energy, and stress levels. Changes in hormone levels can affect how we feel and think, influencing our overall emotional wellbeing.

Genetics: Our genetics can influence how we feel mentally. Knowing about genetic factors, such as the *MTHFR* gene which processes folate (vitamin B9), can help us understand our mental health needs and how to address them.

Substance use: Use of substances such as alcohol and drugs can affect our mental health by altering our brain chemistry and impacting mood, behaviour, and emotional stability. The use of substances, whether occasional or frequent, may influence how we think and feel, and ultimately, our mental health outcomes.

Brain structure and function: Different health behaviours (e.g. poor diet and harmful substance use) can impact mental health by changing the size and activity of brain regions. For example, poor diet can increase the size of the amygdala increasing its sensitivity.

Gut health: I'm sure many of you have heard of the gut–brain relationship. Our gut health determines our gut bacteria, which influences neurotransmitter production and inflammation, impacting brain signals and mood.

Health state: Our physical and mental health are closely connected. When there are changes in one, we will almost always see changes in the other. Any health condition we have will impact our brain function, energy levels, and mood.

Prenatal and early life factors: Early life and prenatal factors can influence our mental health by affecting gene expression, brain development, and the stress response system (hypothalamic–pituitary–adrenal axis). Prenatal stress, nutrition, and caregiving shape neural circuits, emotional regulation, and immune system programming, impacting mental health outcomes.

Immune system function: Our immune system affects our mental health through cytokines, which influence neurotransmitters and neural circuits, contributing to mood, cognition, and behaviour. Inflammation and immune responses can alter neurotransmitter function, stress responses, and neuroplasticity, impacting mental health outcomes.

Exposure to pollutants: Our exposure to air and water pollutants (e.g. pesticides) and heavy metals (e.g. arsenic) impacts neurotransmitter and other functions related to our mental health.

What psychological factors impact our mental health?

Psychological factors are all about how we think, feel, and behave. They can influence our mental health, especially when life throws us curveballs. Let's breakdown some of the common psychological influences that can impact our mental health:

Thoughts: Our thoughts (positive or negative) shape our emotions, guide our actions, and affect how we handle stress. Our expectations and self-esteem also play a role in our mental health satisfaction and overall mood.

Feelings: How we cope with stress or identify, understand, and manage our emotions, or any use of unhealthy coping methods (e.g. avoiding problems or harmful substance use) can significantly influence our mental health.

Actions: The choices we make about what we eat, how much we move, and how well we sleep can all play a part in our mental wellbeing and even create a cycle in which the experience of mental health and lifestyle choices feed into each other.

Stress levels: Our workload, level of engagement in self-care, and coping mechanisms impact our stress levels, which can change the structure of our brain involved in mood (the amygdala) and ultimately how this area of the brain works.

Personality: Some personality traits and individual differences (e.g. level of resilience) influence our susceptibility to stress and mental health problems.

Our past: Life events, especially when we are young, can leave a lasting mark on our mental health.

What social factors impact our mental health?

Social factors are all about the world we live in—things such as the stress we deal with, our financial situation, and the support we get from others. These factors can really impact our mental health, putting extra pressure on us both physically and mentally. They don't act in isolation; they interact with our biology and how we think and feel, affecting how mental health issues can start, continue, or get worse. Let's look at some common social influences on mental health:

Socioeconomic factors: Our income, education, job, and access to services such as healthcare and other resources and opportunities play key roles in wellbeing.

Sense of community: Our community ties and friend and family relationships, including interactions and levels of support, play key roles in our wellbeing and resilience.

Social support: Our support network, in the form of social connections and relationships, contributes to our overall mental wellbeing. The nature of these connections can affect how we feel and function emotionally.

Cultural factors: Our cultural beliefs and practices influence our mental health by shaping attitudes and behaviours related to wellbeing. These perspectives can affect how we approach and manage our mental health.

Life events: How we handle life changes and challenges, such as personal growth from major events, and stress management and coping strategies contribute to our mental health outcomes.

Exposure to discrimination and prejudice: Inclusivity and understanding in an environment can influence mental health and contribute to our sense of belonging.

Social media use: Social media can be a valuable tool for connection and support. How we use social media can impact our mental health (i.e. overuse and exposure to negative material vs healthy use of positive material).

Physical environment: Our living environment, including air, water, and access to green spaces, influences our lifestyle and ultimately our mental health.

The 4-P model

We're going to dive into the 4-P model to understand mental health better. This method helps mental health professionals figure out what affects our mental wellbeing. Here's a quick breakdown of the 4 Ps:

- **Predisposing:** These are factors that make us more vulnerable, such as our genes, early life experiences, or personality traits.
- **Precipitating:** These are triggers or events that can set off mental health issues, such as stressful life events, trauma, or big changes.
- **Perpetuating:** These are things that keep problems going, such as ongoing stress, poor coping strategies, or negative thought patterns.
- **Protective:** These are things that help reduce risks, such as strong social support, good coping skills, and positive experiences.

This model helps us see how different factors interact with our mental health.

How do I boost my mental health?

To simplify, improving our mental wellness means focusing on boosting protective factors as much as possible. This way, we can balance out the effects of any risk factors (such as predisposing, precipitating, and perpetuating factors).

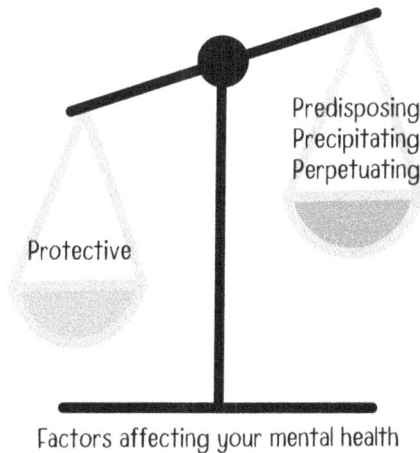

Predisposing
Precipitating
Perpetuating

Protective

Factors affecting your mental health

The more protective factors you add to your life, the better your mental health can become. By actively engaging in positive habits, you strengthen the protective side, which helps counteract risk factors and boosts your mental wellbeing. By contrast, ignoring these protective measures can make you more vulnerable to mental health problems.

Each step in this guide is based on research and is designed to maximise your protective factors, helping you achieve and maintain good mental health.

Now that you have a better understanding of what affects your mental health, you're ready to dive into the common symptoms of mental health issues. Next up, you'll use the checklist to get a sense of your current mental state.

Symptom Checklist

Matt Haig, a mental health advocate and author, wisely said, *"Mental health symptoms don't define who you are. They're something you experience, like rain. You feel it, but you're not the rain."* This means that challenging symptoms are just things you're experiencing, not who you are.

As you start with this guide, first identify and understand the symptoms you're experiencing and their intensity. Having symptoms doesn't necessarily mean you have a mental health condition, but it's a good idea to discuss them with your healthcare provider.

We'll use a checklist of symptoms of common mental health diagnoses from the American Psychiatric Association.

How do mental health symptoms impact your mental health?

Mental health symptoms can show up in different ways and really affect your life and overall wellbeing. They can be grouped into 4 main areas:

EMOTIONAL	COGNITIVE
• persistent feeling of sadness or hopelessness • excessive anxiety • worry, fear, or panic about everyday situations • extreme changes in mood from high to low	• difficulties concentrating, sustaining attention on tasks, and focusing • memory problems, forgetfulness and difficulty remembering important information • difficulties making decisions or feeling overwhelmed by choices
BEHAVIOURAL	PHYSICAL
• withdrawal by avoiding social interactions and activities that were previously enjoyed • changes in eating and sleeping habits • significant weight changes • insomnia or excessive sleep • substance use	• fatigue • chronic tiredness • lack of energy • unexplained aches and pains • headaches • stomach aches • neglecting personal hygiene or appearance

Spotting these symptoms early is key to getting the right help and improving your mental health.

Symptom checklist

Now, let's check in on your current mental state. Use the scale that follows, where 0 means "never" and 4 means "always". Circle the number that best matches how you feel for each item in the table. Then, add up all your numbers to get a total score.

Make sure to record your scores and the date so you can compare them when you use the checklist again in the future.

Likert scale responses key:

0 = Never
1 = Rarely
2 = Sometimes
3 = Regularly
4 = Always

Symptoms	Response
For the past few months, I've been feeling really anxious and constantly worrying about a lot of different things going on in my life.	0 1 2 3 4
I find it really hard to stop worrying once I start.	0 1 2 3 4
For the past few months, I've often felt restless, tense, and like I'm on edge.	0 1 2 3 4
For the past few months, I've been getting tired really easily.	0 1 2 3 4
For the past few months, I've been having a hard time concentrating.	0 1 2 3 4
For the past few months, I've frequently felt pretty irritable.	0 1 2 3 4
For the past few months, I've often felt a lot of muscle tension.	0 1 2 3 4
For the past few months, my sleep has often been really disrupted.	0 1 2 3 4
My anxiety, worry, and physical symptoms have caused me a lot of distress and have really affected important parts of my life, such as my work.	0 1 2 3 4
For the past 2 weeks, I've often felt down most of the day, almost every day, like I'm sad, empty, or hopeless.	0 1 2 3 4

For the past 2 weeks, I've noticed that I've lost a lot of interest or enjoyment in almost everything I used to do, and it's been like that most of the day, nearly every day.	0 1 2 3 4
For the past 2 weeks, I've had noticeable weight changes, either losing weight without trying or gaining weight, with a shift of more than 5% of my body weight in a month. My appetite has also changed significantly, almost every day.	0 1 2 3 4
For the past 2 weeks, I've been dealing with either trouble sleeping or sleeping too much, almost every day.	0 1 2 3 4
For the past 2 weeks, I've often felt either really restless or unusually slowed down, almost every day.	0 1 2 3 4
For the past 2 weeks, I've felt drained or low on energy almost every day.	0 1 2 3 4
For the past 2 weeks, I've been feeling worthless or dealing with a lot of excessive or misplaced guilt almost every day.	0 1 2 3 4
For the past 2 weeks, I've had a hard time focusing or making decisions almost every day.	0 1 2 3 4
For the past 2 weeks, I've been having recurring thoughts about death (not just being afraid of dying), and I've also had thoughts about suicide without a specific plan, or I've made a suicide attempt or had a specific plan.	0 1 2 3 4
My symptoms are causing me a lot of distress and are really affecting my social life, work, and other important areas of my life.	0 1 2 3 4
Total:	

How do I interpret my checklist results?

You should now have a clearer understanding of the symptoms you might be experiencing and how intense they are. The maximum possible score on the checklist is 76. Here's a quick guide to help you interpret your total score:

- **No symptoms:** 0
- **Mild symptoms:** 1–19
- **Moderate symptoms:** 20–38
- **Severe symptoms:** 39–76

For example, if you scored 3 for each item on the checklist, your total would be 57, which falls into the severe range. On the other hand, a total score between 1 and 19 suggests mild symptoms, while a score between 20 and 38 indicates moderate symptoms. If your score is 39 or higher, it points to more severe symptoms.

If your score falls into the mild range or above, it's a good idea to set up an appointment with a general practitioner, psychologist, or mental health professional to talk more about your symptoms. If your score is in the moderate or severe range, it's important to prioritise this appointment.

If you answered anything other than 0 (never) on the checklist item assessing thoughts about death and suicide, reach out to someone you trust and make an urgent appointment with a mental health professional. If you're having current thoughts of suicide, go to the nearest hospital emergency room right away for immediate support.

After completing the 10 steps in this guide, use the checklist again to see how your results have changed. Keep in mind that progress can be gradual and might show up as small improvements over time.

How do I improve my current mental health state?

Now that you have a clear picture of your current mental health symptoms, you're ready to begin step one of this guide. Each step and checklist is here to help you tackle these symptoms. By following each step, you'll work towards reducing the severity of your symptoms and improving your overall mental health.

Step One: Health Screening

In this section, we'll cover the most common health conditions and deficiencies that can impact your mental wellbeing. We'll also go over which health screenings you should get and explain the difference between "normal" and "optimal" results when it comes to mental health.

Dr Charles Gant, a medical doctor who takes a holistic approach to health, has a powerful saying: *"Unless you test, you've guessed!"*

Right now, the way mental health is treated is often pretty guesswork based. Doctors might see your symptoms and jump straight to prescribing antidepressants without running any formal tests. It's only if you go to a holistic doctor that you might get some blood work done for things like vitamin D or thyroid levels. It's pretty wild when you think about it.

Imagine if an oncologist just assumed you had cancer because of some symptoms and started you on chemotherapy without doing proper tests like blood work, imaging, or biopsies. That would be absurd, right? It's the same with mental health. You could be dealing with symptoms that are actually signs of an underlying issue or deficiency that's never been properly diagnosed. It's like trying to solve a puzzle without all the pieces—you might be missing a big part of the picture.

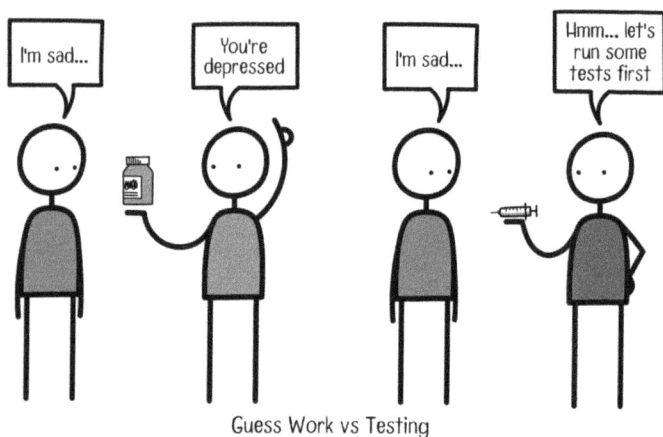

Guess Work vs Testing

If you've noticed any mental health symptoms that you'd rather not be dealing with, it's a good idea to get a range of health screening tests done. These tests can help identify if any common health issues or deficiencies might be affecting your mental health. Catching these issues early means you can address them right away and potentially avoid unnecessary treatments. For instance, if you're feeling down and get diagnosed with depression, having done some initial health screenings might have revealed a vitamin D deficiency. Fixing that with a simple supplement could lift your mood and avoid a depression diagnosis altogether. Many medications, including antidepressants, can also unintentionally deplete important nutrients and minerals, increasing your risk of deficiencies.

Make sure to ask for a printed copy of your test results so you can compare them to the optimal ranges we'll discuss later. This is crucial because ***many health providers don't always flag borderline results, but fixing these can sometimes make a big difference to your mental health***.

Be aware that some general practitioners might skip certain tests because of their cost. If that happens, you can ask to pay for these tests out-of-pocket if it's feasible for you. I've also listed the tests in order of their importance for mental health, so you know which ones to prioritise if you're on a budget.

How will normal vs optimal results impact my mental health?

Have you ever had blood tests where everything came back "normal", but you still felt off? That's because normal ranges from lab tests can be quite broad. Just because something falls within the lab's range doesn't mean it's ideal for your health. It is important to understand that *normal is not optimal*.

- **Abnormal results:** If your results fall here, it means these are values outside the "normal" range, indicating potential deficiencies or problems that will almost certainly negatively impact your mental health.

- **Normal results:** These are values that fall within the range considered typical for a generally healthy population relatively free of major disease. Labs determine this range by analysing results from a large group of mostly healthy people. If your results fall within this range, you can still experience mental health problems because this doesn't always reflect the best possible health.

- **Optimal results:** These are specific values within the normal range that are linked to the best mental health outcomes. They're based on clinical guidelines or research and are more tailored to ideal functioning than to just avoiding disease. Optimal ranges might vary based on factors such as age, sex, and overall health.

Case study:

A few years ago, out of the blue, I started feeling tired, had brain fog, and wasn't sleeping well. I got a bunch of blood tests done, including one for vitamin D, and everything came back as "normal". But when I looked closer, I saw that my vitamin D level was 53 nmol/L. Even though this was within the lab's "normal" range (50 to 125 nmol/L), it's not considered ideal for good health, which is usually 100 nmol/L. So, I decided to improve my vitamin D levels with some changes to my diet and by taking supplements. When I got tested again, my level was up to 90 nmol/L, and all my symptoms had gone away.

What are the optimal results for mental wellness?

There are many different health screening domains that can impact mental health, but we're focusing on the ones that are most critical. Most of these tests involve blood work, but some might also need saliva or stool samples. Getting these tests done can help you identify any health issues that might be affecting your mental wellbeing, so you can address them and reduce their impact.

In the table that follows, you'll find a list of recommended screening tests ranked by their importance (vitamin D, for example, is at the top because it's particularly crucial). The table also shows the optimal results for each test in terms of mental health. Make sure to get a printed copy of your results so you can fill them in on the table and compare them with the optimal ranges provided.

Keep in mind that the optimal results listed are based on healthy adults who are at least 18 years old.

Labs around the world might use different units of measurement for tests. I've included the most common units here for your convenience, but if your lab results are in a different unit, you can use online converters or ask your lab or doctor to provide them in the units you prefer.

If you need to calculate optimal results based on a percentage of the lab's 'normal' range, here's an example:

- **Optimal result:** In the top 20% of your lab's normal range
- **Example normal lab range:** 200 to 700 pg/ml
- **Find the total range:** 700 (top of lab range) - 200 (bottom of lab range) = 500
- **Calculate 20% of the range:** 500 x 0.2 = 100
- **Determine the starting point for the top 20%:** Subtract 100 from the top of the range (700) = 600
- **Optimal range:** 600 – 700 pg/ml

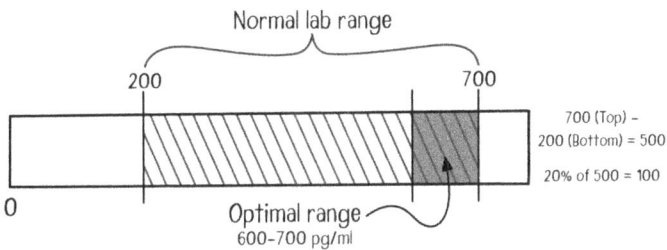

Following the table, I've provided more detailed information on each test if you want to understand why they're important. If you're not interested, feel free to skip ahead.

Test	Optimal results	Result	Date
Vitamin D	Close to 100 nmol/L		
Active vitamin B12	Close to 125 pmol/L		
Folate (B9)	Close to 35 nmol/L		

Test	Optimal results	Result	Date
Homocysteine	Below 7 µmol/L		
Omega-3	Between 10 and 12%		
hsCRP	Below 1 mg/L		
TSH (thyroid)	Close to 1 mU/L		
T3 and T4 (thyroid)	In the top 20% of your lab's normal range		
Ferritin (iron)	Close to 150 ug/L		
Glucose	In the bottom 20% of your lab's normal range		
Magnesium (RBC)	In the top 20% of your lab's normal range		
ALT and AST (liver)	In the bottom 50% of your lab's normal range		
Bilirubin (liver)	In the middle 50% of lab's normal range		
Electrolyte panel	In the normal lab range (outside of limits)		
Morning cortisol	In the normal lab range (outside of limits)		
Evening cortisol	In the bottom 50% of your lab's normal range		
Cytokine panel	In the normal lab range (outside of limits)		
Zinc	In the top 20% of your lab's normal range		
Sex hormones	In the normal lab range (outside of limits)		
Neurotransmitters	In the normal lab range (outside of limits)		

Test	Optimal results	Result	Date
Celiac disease panel	Negative result		
MTHFR gene	Negative result		

Note. Abbreviations and units used in the table are defined as follows:

ALT: Alanine aminotransferase

AST: Aspartate aminotransferase

hsCRP: High-sensitivity C-reactive protein

mg/L: Milligrams per litre

MTHFR **gene:** Methylenetetrahydrofolate reductase gene

mU/L: Milliunits per litre

nmol/L: Nanomoles per litre

pmol/L: Picomoles per litre

RBC: Red blood cells

T3: Triiodothyronine

T4: Thyroxine

TSH: Thyroid-stimulating hormone

µg/L: Micrograms per litre

µmol/L: Micromoles per litre

1. Vitamin D overview

Vitamin D is *the only vitamin our bodies can produce on their own with the help of direct sunlight.* Ask yourself, "Why are our bodies designed to make their own vitamin D?" Some argue this is due to this vitamin being the most important for our health. For our bodies to produce their own vitamin D, we need direct skin-to-sunlight contact without window or clothing barriers. Vitamin D can be stored long-term in the body and takes time to accumulate.

Vitamin D benefits our wellbeing by supporting neurotransmitter production, reducing inflammation, regulating stress responses, and protecting brain function. It might surprise you, but 2023 research led by Aiyong Cui involving 7.9 million people found that *half of us* don't have enough vitamin D; low levels, according to a study led by Şerife Akpınar, are linked with increased mental health symptoms.

Low vitamin D can cause:

- persistent tiredness and low energy
- mood swings and sadness
- worry, nervousness, and panic attacks
- difficulty concentrating and memory impairment
- sleep disturbances.

2. Active vitamin B12 (holotranscobalamin or HoloTC) overview

Two types of vitamin B12 exist: total B12 and active B12 (also called HoloTC). Standard practice is to first assess total B12. However, *ask for the active B12 (HoloTC) form to be tested instead* as this is far more important for mental health.

A 4-year study from the University of Limerick, led by Eamon Laird, found that people low in vitamin B12 have a *51% higher risk of mental health issues.* The good news is this deficiency is often reversible, according to research led by Tan Yongjun from Chongqing Medical University among 38,000 people.

Vitamin B12 is crucial for mental health—it helps produce neurotransmitters, keeps nerves and cells healthy, supports red blood cell and DNA formation, boosts energy, and regulates sleep and stress. According to Professor Regan Bailey's research, about 1 in 4 Americans are low in vitamin B12, based on a national survey. If you're feeling off, checking your B12 levels might be a good idea!

Low vitamin B12 can cause:

- fatigue and depression

- anxiety, nervousness and panic attacks
- irritability
- poor concentration and memory
- disrupted sleep.

3. Folate (vitamin B9) overview

Ansley Bender and colleagues from the University of South Florida found that people with mental health challenges often have lower folate levels in their blood and eat less folate compared with those without such challenges. Folate is important because it helps make deoxyribonucleic acid (DNA) and ribonucleic acid (RNA), process proteins, keep nerves healthy, and produce neurotransmitters and energy. Dr Rogers from the World Health Organization discovered that at least *1 in 4 people globally* have low folate levels.

Low folate can cause:

- fatigue and brain fog
- depression
- irritability and mood swings
- anxiety
- poor sleep.

4. Homocysteine overview

Homocysteine is an amino acid found in the blood. Maintaining optimal homocysteine levels supports your body's conversion of unusable, inactive B vitamins to usable, active forms, which is vital for producing mood-regulating neurotransmitters (i.e. serotonin, dopamine, and norepinephrine). An estimated *10% to 20% of us* have high homocysteine levels.

High homocysteine can cause:

- memory problems
- inflammation

- depression
- impaired neurotransmitter synthesis
- fatigue
- irritability.

5. Omega-3 overview

Most people don't get enough omega-3 fatty acids, so *omega-3 deficiency is quite common.* The main types are eicosapentaenoic acid (EPA) and docosahexaenoic acid (DHA), which come from fish, and ALA, found in certain algae. Omega-3s support brain cell growth, help neurotransmitters work, improve brain flexibility, and regulate mood. To check your omega-3 levels, a screening looks at EPA and DHA in your blood cell membranes.

Low omega-3 can cause:

- memory problems
- mood swings
- depression and anxiety
- fatigue and difficulty concentrating
- irritability.

6. High-sensitivity C-reactive protein (hsCRP) overview

About *1 in 5 of us* has high levels of high-sensitivity C-reactive protein (hsCRP), which signals systemic inflammation. Elevated hsCRP means there's a lot of inflammation in both the body and brain, which can negatively affect mental health.

High hsCRP can cause:

- sleep problems and fatigue
- depression
- anxiety
- appetite changes
- muscle tension

- stomach upset.

7. Thyroid (TSH, T3, T4) overview

Dr Ali Alzahrani and colleagues' research suggests that at least 10% of people have thyroid dysfunction, and 60% of them don't even know it. That's around *33 million Americans*, with women being more affected. I can relate to this personally. As a child, I had persistent fatigue and low energy for months. After some blood tests, I was diagnosed with hypothyroidism and got the treatment I needed.

High thyroid can cause:

- anxiety
- increased heart rate
- irritability
- restlessness
- sleep disturbances.

Low thyroid can cause:

- depression
- fatigue
- cognitive slowness
- mood swings.

8. Iron (ferritin) overview

Iron levels are measured using various markers, with ferritin being a key one. Ferritin is a protein that stores iron in the body, so its levels show how much iron is available for use. This makes ferritin especially useful for understanding mental health. Iron is crucial for brain function, because it helps regulate neurotransmitters, produce energy, and supply oxygen-rich blood to the brain. Around *10 million Americans* are iron deficient.

Low iron can cause:

- tiredness
- weakness
- lack of energy
- depression.

9. Blood glucose overview

Glucose is the main energy source for our brains, so imbalances can really affect mental health. Proper blood glucose levels help stabilise mood, improve focus, reduce anxiety, and regulate sleep. Around *10% of us* have issues with our blood glucose levels.

Unstable blood glucose can cause:

- irritability
- anxiety
- depression
- confusion
- fatigue.

10. Magnesium (red blood cell) overview

Magnesium can be measured in different ways, but the magnesium red blood cell (RBC) test gives the most accurate picture of your magnesium levels. This is important for mental health, because magnesium helps regulate sleep, manage stress, support neurotransmitter function, and boost mood. Unfortunately, about *3 out of 4 of us* don't get enough magnesium daily, which raises the risk of deficiency.

Low magnesium can cause:

- anxiety, nervousness, and panic attacks
- depression
- fatigue and low energy
- headaches
- insomnia and sleep challenges.

11. Liver function test (ALT, AST, bilirubin) overview

A liver function test is a blood panel that checks enzymes, proteins, and other substances to assess how well your liver is working. The liver is essential for both physical and mental health, handling over 500 important tasks like detoxifying harmful substances, regulating hormones and neurotransmitters, managing inflammation, and storing key nutrients. People with mental health issues are *much more likely to have abnormal liver function.*

Poor liver function can cause:

- mood swings
- brain fog
- depression and anxiety
- sleep challenges.

12. Electrolytes overview

Electrolytes are essential minerals such as sodium, potassium, calcium, chloride, magnesium, phosphate, and bicarbonate. They play a crucial role in boosting serotonin, stabilising mood, reducing stress and anxiety, promoting sleep, maintaining fluid balance in our cells, and coordinating chemical reactions in the body. While it's hard to pin down exactly how common electrolyte imbalances are, we know they occur relatively frequently.

Unstable electrolytes can cause:

- mood swings
- confusion
- anxiety, racing heart, and panic attacks
- fatigue.

13. Cortisol overview

Diagnosing cortisol dysregulation can be tricky. Typically, it involves a blood test and a take-home saliva test that you do yourself in the morning and evening. It's normal for cortisol levels to fluctuate throughout the day. Cortisol is a hormone produced by the adrenal glands and is crucial for managing stress.

Dr Nader Salari and colleagues' research shows that about *1 in 3* regularly experience chronic stress, which can throw off cortisol levels. Additionally, Ewelina Dziurkowska from the Medical University of Gdansk found that *half of those diagnosed with depression* also have cortisol problems.

Low cortisol can cause:

- fatigue and low energy
- mood swings and irritability
- difficulty coping with stress
- brain fog.

High cortisol can cause:

- anxiety and nervousness
- depression
- difficulty sleeping
- decreased motivation.

14. Cytokine overview

Cytokines are small proteins released by our cells, especially those in the immune system. They play a key role in controlling inflammation, immune responses, and cell communication. Balancing cytokine activity is important for regulating mood, managing stress, sleep, and cognitive performance. Keeping them in check might even lead to new ways to manage mental health symptoms.

High cytokine levels can cause:

- mood disorders
- difficulty with concentration and memory

- fatigue
- sleep disturbances.

Low cytokine levels can cause:

- fatigue
- mood swings and depression
- increased sensitivity to stress
- cognitive difficulties.

15. Zinc overview

Mild zinc deficiencies can be hard to spot with blood tests, which is why zinc testing is often not a top priority. Zinc is important for our immune system, DNA production, sleep, and neurotransmitter function. Around *2 billion people globally are zinc deficient.*

Low zinc can cause:

- depression
- anxiety
- emotional instability
- cognitive difficulties.

16. Sex hormones (testosterone and estradiol) overview

Testosterone is a steroid hormone mainly produced in the testes and ovaries, with smaller amounts coming from the adrenal glands in all genders. Estradiol, a key female sex hormone, is also present in all genders. Both testosterone and estradiol help with mood stability, neurotransmitter regulation, and overall emotional wellbeing.

Low sex hormone levels can cause:

- depression
- anxiety
- cognitive decline

- mood swings
- fatigue.

High sex hormone levels can cause:

- mood swings
- aggression
- irritability
- anxiety
- impulsivity.

17. Neurotransmitter advanced profile overview

A neurotransmitter profile measures levels of important chemicals like serotonin, dopamine, and norepinephrine. These neurotransmitters are crucial for mood stability, cognitive function, stress and anxiety management, sleep, motivation, energy, and appetite. Knowing your neurotransmitter profile can help guide treatment choices, including the use of antidepressants.

Low neurotransmitter levels can cause:

- depression
- anxiety
- fatigue and low energy
- irritability and mood swings
- sleep disturbances.

18. Coeliac disease panel overview

A positive coeliac disease panel means you have gluten intolerance, which can cause inflammation that disrupts the gut–brain connection. If you have coeliac disease, following a gluten-free diet can help ease symptoms and boost mental wellbeing, leading to better overall health and quality of life.

Coeliac disease can cause:

- anxiety

- depression
- irritability and mood swings
- brain fog and lethargy
- sleep disturbances.

19. MTHFR gene overview

Dr Will Cole, a functional medicine doctor, found that *up to 40% of people have an MTHFR gene mutation*. This mutation can affect mental health by impairing the body's ability to process folate and vitamin B12. As a result, it can lead to high homocysteine levels and a lack of the activated forms of folate and vitamin B12 that our bodies need.

MTHFR gene mutation can cause:

- anxiety
- depression
- irritability and mood swings
- brain fog and fatigue
- sleep disturbances.

Case study:

A close friend of mine—let's call her Stacey—came to me with a bunch of mental health symptoms, but she couldn't pinpoint any specific triggers. Everything in her life seemed to be going well except for these symptoms. I suggested she get a few tests done, including the ones listed in this step. The results gave us an immediate answer: she was severely deficient in vitamin D and active B12 and had low iron levels. Stacey was surprised because she thought her nutritious diet and healthy lifestyle would have prevented this. After a few months of targeted supplementation, she was able to reverse these deficiencies, and her symptoms disappeared.

How do I improve my health screening results?

Getting thorough health screenings is a great way to figure out what might be affecting your mental health. If you get your levels in the optimal ranges, it can really help improve your symptoms and set you on a path to feeling better. If some results aren't quite where they should be, plan to check them again in about 3 to 6 months.

1. Get a copy: Always ask for a copy of your health and screening results to take home. It's important to have this information handy.

2. Review your results: Compare your results with the optimal ranges mentioned in this guide and note any areas that are off.

3. Use targeted supplements: Start taking the supplements we discuss in the next step to address any areas where your screening results need improvement.

4. Focus on nutrition: Follow the nutrition tips later in this guide to boost your intake of foods that improve your screening results but also reduce the impact of nutritional choices that detract or worsen screening domains.

5. Complete the guide: As you go through the rest of this guide, you'll find steps that'll help improve your screening results, such as getting better sleep to lower inflammation.

6. Rescreen in 3–6 months: After finishing this guide and giving it 3 to 6 months, get those areas that were out of range tested again to check your progress.

Step One Checklist: Health Screening

You've got a good understanding of how certain health issues can mimic mental health problems, and you know how your screening results compare to the ideal. Now, use this checklist to make sure you're getting the most out of this information:

☐ **Review the health screening content:** Go through the screening details and make sure you understand the concepts. It's important that you're comfortable with this step.

☐ **Complete the tests:** Complete each of the screening tests recommended in this step.

☐ **Get a printout copy:** Ask for take-home copies of all the health screening tests you've done.

☐ **Compare your results:** Use the table in this step to see how your screening results measure up to the optimal levels.

☐ **Note any differences:** If your results are significantly different from the optimal ranges, it might be a good idea to consult with a functional practitioner. They look at your whole health picture to help find solutions.

☐ **Move on:** Once you're done with this step, proceed to the targeted supplementation step of the guide.

☐ **Plan for rescreening:** Set a reminder to redo these screenings about 3 months after you've followed the guide.

Step Two: Targeted Supplementation

In this section, I'll give you a clear overview of some of the most researched supplements for boosting mental wellbeing. I'll cover which supplements have strong safety profiles, their recommended dosages, and the best forms to use for optimal results.

Before you start taking any of these supplements, it's crucial to consult with your general practitioner. This step is important to ensure that the supplements are safe for you and compatible with your individual health needs.

Just to clarify, when I mention supplementation here, I'm not talking about just grabbing any vitamins or tablets you find. Instead, I'm referring to adding specific vitamins, minerals, and nutrients in a targeted way to enhance your overall health and mental wellbeing.

Targeted supplementation can be a strategic tool for mental health. It helps address nutritional gaps, reduce inflammation, and support neurotransmitter and hormone balance, which in turn supports cognitive function, mood stability, and overall emotional health.

I should mention that I personally take every supplement listed in this step and have seen significant benefits from them.

Targeted supplementation is one of the first practical steps in this guide because it helps you actively manage your psychological wellbeing, fostering a sense of empowerment and control over your own mental health. This approach not only aids in symptom management but also supports long-term brain health and cognitive vitality, laying a strong foundation for sustained emotional wellbeing.

In today's flood of information about dietary supplements, you've probably encountered a wide range of opinions on their benefits and drawbacks. The good news is that research is growing, and the evidence supporting certain supplements and dosages is becoming increasingly strong, and in some cases, impossible to disregard. *However, it's important to be aware that some supplements can contain potentially harmful or ineffective ingredients such as genetically modified organisms, artificial flavours, soy, maltodextrin or gluten. Others might have less bioavailable forms that are poorly absorbed or dosages that are too low to make a real difference.*

Here's the key takeaway: ***Only a small percentage of supplements on the market are free from harmful ingredients, offer dosages proven to support mental health, and come in forms that your body can effectively use.*** I'll go into more detail on this in the pages that follow, but the main point is to do your research and choose wisely to avoid wasting time and money.

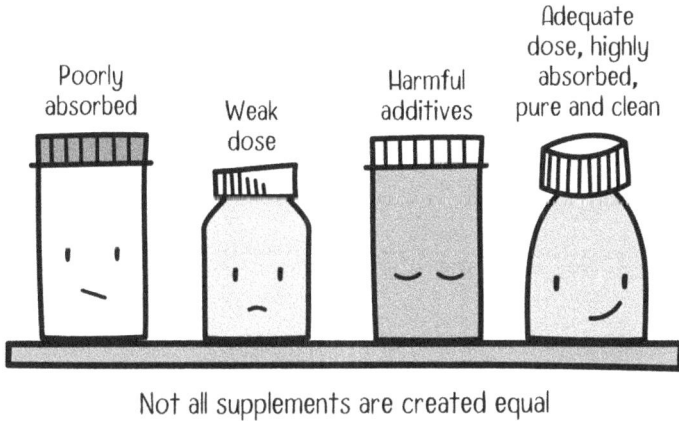

Not all supplements are created equal

How will targeted supplementation boost my mental health?

Targeted supplementation can do more than just fill specific nutrient gaps—it can actually support neurotransmitter production, reduce inflammation, and enhance brain function. This approach can lead to a better mood, decreased anxiety and depression, and overall improved brain health and stress resilience.

Neurotransmitter synthesis: Certain vitamins and minerals in the supplements I recommend are key to making mood-related neurotransmitters, so taking supplements can help make sure you have enough of these nutrients to produce them. For instance, B vitamins, such as B6, B12, and folate, are essential for creating neurotransmitters that regulate mood, such as serotonin and dopamine.

Anti-inflammatory: Reducing inflammation promotes mental health. Most supplements I recommend here have this effect; for example, the omega-3 fatty acids in fish oil supplements directly reduce brain inflammation caused by lifestyle factors (e.g. stress and poor diet).

Antioxidant protection: Many of the supplements recommended here help protect against stress and damage to your cells (oxidative stress) by supporting your body's antioxidant defence system. For instance, vitamin C acts as an antioxidant that shields your brain cells from stress and damage.

Hormone regulation: Every supplement recommended in this step benefits your hormones in some way. For example, vitamin D plays a role in regulating mood and warding off depression by influencing the production of hormones such as cortisol and thyroid. It also has receptors in brain areas involved in mood regulation.

Energy production: One of the most common signs of poor mental health is feeling tired, low on energy, and just plain worn out. The supplements in this step all help boost your energy levels. For example, an active B complex gives your body a direct energy boost—it's the same stuff you find in energy tablets and hangover relief drinks, which should give you an idea of how effective it can be.

Enhanced gut–brain axis: Gut health is important for your mental wellbeing. The supplements in this step are all designed to support and improve your gut health. For instance, fish oil helps balance your good gut bacteria, keeps your gut lining strong, and supports your immune system.

Improved sleep: Sleep is essential for your mental health, and the supplements listed in this step all help improve sleep in some way. For example, magnesium glycinate is often used as a sleep aid to boost both the quality and amount of sleep you get.

Reducing stress: Stress is often the first trigger for mental health issues. The supplements in this step all help reduce stress in different ways. For example, magnesium plays a role in over 300 processes in the body, many of which are linked to how your body handles stress.

What supplements should I take for my mental health?

Before you start taking any supplements, it's always a good idea to check with a healthcare professional to make sure they're safe for you and your specific needs. Do not exceed any of the upper limits I have mentioned in the supplement criteria and directions for use for each supplement type, as this can lead to unwanted side effects.

I've ranked the recommended supplements in order of importance. If you're on a budget and can only get one or two, focus on the top two: vitamin D and omega-3 fatty acids. Even though there are thousands of supplements out there, only a few have a significant impact on mental health.

You might have heard about other supplements for mental health, such as St John's wort, but this list only includes those with the highest safety standards. When it comes to supplements, quality matters a lot. The best, most effective options often cost more, which can make them less accessible for everyone.

1. Vitamin D3 (with K2)

If you need convincing, consider this: vitamin D is the **only** vitamin our bodies can produce on their own. Ever wonder why our bodies are designed to make this vitamin but not others? To produce vitamin D, you need direct sunlight on your skin, without anything blocking it, such as windows or clothes. Supplementing might be especially important if you live in a cooler climate, work indoors, or are heading into the winter months.

Vitamin D tops the list because there's strong evidence that it plays a key role in mental health. For instance, research from the Center for Biological Sciences in Brazil, led by Dr Gleicilaine Casseb, found that vitamin D supplements are linked to reduced symptoms of depression and anxiety.

Supplement criteria: When looking for a vitamin D supplement, choose one that contains both *1,000 IU (25 mcg)* *of vitamin D3 and around 100 mcg of vitamin K2.* K2 helps absorb vitamin D and direct it to the right places.

Case study:

Let me tell you about Emma. Every winter, Emma's mood would drop, no matter how much she exercised, ate well, or tried to get outside. Nothing seemed to help with her winter blues. I mentioned that low vitamin D levels could contribute to seasonal depression and suggested she get a blood test. The test showed her vitamin D levels were low, so I recommended she take a supplement for the rest of the winter. After just a few weeks, Emma noticed a real difference: her mood improved, she had more energy, and she felt more optimistic. For the first time in years, winter didn't feel so tough.

Directions for use: Get a blood test before starting vitamin D. If your levels are below 80 nmol/L, consider supplementing with 25 mcg daily; *if they're 100 nmol/L or higher, do not supplement*. Many people are deficient, so chances are you'll be below 80 nmol/L. It can take about a month of daily use to see changes. After 1 to 3 months, retest to determine whether you should continue. For best results, take vitamin D in the morning with your first meal.

2. Omega-3 fatty acids

I've been taking an omega-3 fish oil supplement every day for the last 10 years, and it's made a big difference for me. If you haven't heard of blue zones, you should check them out! These are places around the world where people live much longer and healthier lives than average. One of the secrets to their longevity is eating a lot of fish, which is packed with omega-3 fatty acids.

Research from the University of Cincinnati, led by Professor Robert McNamara, found that regularly consuming omega-3s, such as EPA and DHA, can reduce the risk of mental health issues and improve mood. People in the blue zones usually have higher levels of these omega-3s, and studies show that those with higher omega-3 levels in their blood often experience better mental health and fewer mental health issues.

Supplementing with EPA and DHA doesn't just help with mood, it can also boost the effectiveness of antidepressant medications. Since our bodies can't make these fatty acids on their own and most of us don't eat enough fish, taking a supplement can be crucial for maintaining good mental health.

Supplement criteria: Research from the Chinese Center for Chronic Disease Control, led by Yuhua Liao, looked at 26 different studies and found that, for the best mental health benefits, you should aim for at least 1 gram of omega-3s a day. Make sure your supplement has more EPA than DHA—ideally, at least 60% EPA. For example, my omega-3 supplement has 320 mg of EPA and 210 mg of DHA per capsule. I take 2 capsules daily, which gives me 640 mg of EPA and 420 mg of DHA.

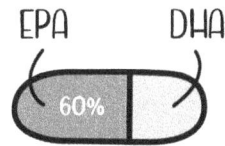

When choosing a supplement, make sure it's tested and certified to be low in harmful substances such as lead, mercury, and poly-chlorinated biphenyls (PCBs). My fish oil supplement even has a chart on the label showing it's well below safety limits for these toxins.

If you're not into fish oil, there are also omega-3 supplements made from algae that provide both EPA and DHA.

Case study:

After experiencing unexplained mental health symptoms, Emily took my recommendation to test her omega-3 levels. The results showed only 3%, about a third of the optimal level. I suggested she start taking a fish oil supplement.

Within a couple of months, Emily began noticing subtle but positive changes in her mental health. Her mood improved, she felt more focused, and her overall mental clarity increased, showing the impact of addressing the deficiency.

Directions for use: Make sure you're getting 1 gram of combined EPA and DHA daily—not just 1 gram of fish oil. For instance, each of my fish oil capsules is 1 gram but only has 320 mg of EPA and 210 mg of DHA, which adds up to 530 mg of EPA and DHA combined. So, I take 2 capsules a day to get a total of 1.06 grams of actual EPA and DHA.

This is key because the mental health benefits from fish oil usually start with a daily dose of at least 1 gram of combined EPA and DHA. Remember, it can take up to 3 months for EPA and DHA to build up in your brain and up to 6 months to see improvements in mood. Omega-3 supplements are a long-term commitment, not a quick fix, so make sure to take your fish oil daily with your first meal and stay consistent.

3. Active (vitamin) B complex

Dr Uma Naidoo, a nutritional psychiatrist and brain expert at Harvard Medical School, stresses that B vitamins are *the most important for our brain's health.* That's why they're third on our list of recommended supplements. Research backs this up: Brazilian biomedical scientists Jaqueline Borges-Vieira and Camila Souza Cardoso reviewed 20 high-quality studies and found that taking B vitamins can effectively help improve symptoms of depression and anxiety.

A typical B vitamin complex includes all 8 essential B vitamins: B1, B2, B3, B5, B6, B7, B9, and B12. These vitamins are key for energy production, which makes them especially beneficial if you're struggling with low energy and motivation.

Supplement criteria: B vitamin supplements are often available in inactive forms, meaning your liver has to convert them into their active, usable state. *Always avoid these versions*. To prevent putting extra strain on your liver, choose activated B vitamins, which your body can use immediately.

For example, some B complex supplements use folic acid (an inactive form of B9), while others provide the more effective, active form called 5-MTHF. Choosing an activated B complex ensures the vitamins are ready to work right away.

When selecting a B vitamin supplement, look for one that's free from common allergens, such as eggs, milk, peanuts, gluten, and lactose, and avoid artificial colours, flavours, or preservatives. If you're only supplementing with B12, choose a product that includes both methylcobalamin and adenosylcobalamin. These forms are highly absorbable and work together to maximise their effectiveness.

cyanocobalamin
(synthetic)

methycobalamin and
adenosylcobalamin
(natural)

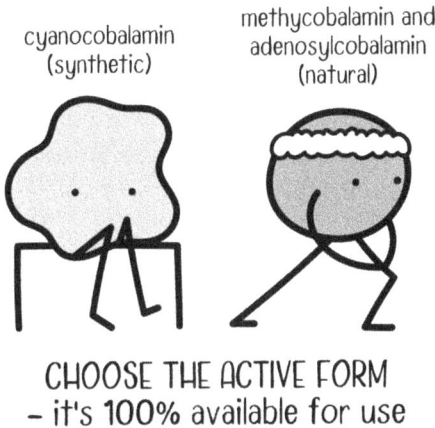

CHOOSE THE ACTIVE FORM
- it's **100%** available for use

Case study:

Dean was living his best life, thriving in his social circle. But one night, while out for dinner, out of nowhere, he began sweating and feeling anxious, and completely lost his appetite halfway through his meal. He shrugged it off at first, but these episodes started happening daily and were identified as panic attacks. I recommended that Dean get his active B12 levels checked through a blood test, which showed a deficiency. I advised him to start taking a daily activated B complex supplement, and within 2 weeks, his anxiety and panic attacks completely disappeared.

Directions for use: Before starting any active B complex supplements, it's a good idea to get a blood test to ensure they're safe for you. Specifically, ask for a test for the active form of B12, holotranscobalamin (HoloTC) for a more accurate reading. If your active B12 or B9 (folate) levels are close to the upper limit of the normal range, use supplements only when needed, such as on particularly stressful days. If your levels are above the normal range, talk to your doctor, who might suggest additional tests, and avoid B vitamin supplements with B9 and/or B12.

B complex supplements will show benefits faster than omega-3s and vitamin D, sometimes within just a few doses. If your B9 or B12 levels are near the upper range, stick to low-dose supplements. For normal levels, you can use them as needed for a mood boost. If your B12 or folate levels are low, try taking 400 mcg daily for 3 months, then retest.

B vitamins are great for turning food into energy and combating fatigue, so it's best to take your B complex in the morning, with or before breakfast. I've noticed that my morning B complex gives me a boost similar to coffee. Just be careful not to take it too late in the day, or it might interfere with your sleep.

4. Magnesium (glycinate or L-threonate)

Most of us don't get enough magnesium daily—about *75% of people are deficient*. Lifestyle factors like stress, caffeine, alcohol, and sugar can lower your magnesium levels. If you need more reasons to consider magnesium, remember it's involved in *over 300 biochemical reactions* in the body, many of which impact mental health. That's why magnesium is a key ingredient in bath salts designed to relieve stress and anxiety!

Research from the University of Leeds, led by Dr Neil Boyle, found that magnesium supplementation can help with anxiety, based on a review of 18 different studies. Similarly, a review of 7 studies from Kashan University of Medical Sciences, led by Mahdi Moabedi, found that magnesium can also benefit those with depression.

Magnesium comes in various forms, each with different mental health benefits. I'll go into more detail about these forms in the supplement criteria that follows.

Supplement criteria: Magnesium comes in different forms, but for mental health, focus on just 2 types. If you're dealing with *anxiety and stress, go with magnesium glycinate*. For *depression and low mood, try magnesium L-threonate*. If you're dealing with both, you can take a lower dose (100–200 mg) of each type together.

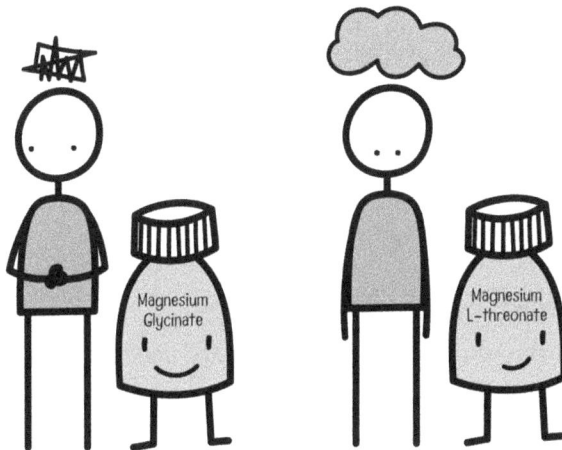

Adults can safely take up to 300 mg of magnesium per day for women and 400 mg for men.

Case study:

Jake had struggled with anxiety for years. Every night, his mind raced, making it nearly impossible to sleep. He'd tried everything—meditation, cutting back on caffeine, even sleep aids—but nothing worked. His anxiety kept him on edge, and his sleepless nights left him exhausted. Jake experimented with different magnesium supplements in the forms of carbonate, oxide, sulfate, and hydroxide, with no luck. After determining Jake had not tried magnesium in the form of glycinate I advised him to try this form. While he hesitated to spend more money to try yet another different form, he gave it a shot and couldn't believe the difference glycinate made for him. After taking his first dose he felt calm, sleep came quickly, and he woke up feeling rested.

Directions for use: My magnesium supplement is 110 mg per capsule. I usually take one right after work, and if it's been a really stressful day, I'll take a second one about 30 minutes before bed. You can adjust when you take it based on your needs. If you often feel anxious at a certain time of day, try taking your first capsule about an hour before that time to help prevent it. For general mood support, taking your supplement in the evening can also help with sleep. You should start to feel some relief within an hour of taking it.

5. Zinc (picolinate or bisglycinate)

Research shows that even a mild zinc deficiency can hurt mental health. One theory is that zinc is essential for serotonin transmission in the brain. Serotonin helps stabilise mood, so zinc plays a big role in keeping you feeling balanced. It's also crucial for neurotransmission and nervous system function, plus it has antioxidant and anti-inflammatory benefits, making it a great all-rounder for mental wellbeing.

If you need more reasons to consider zinc, doctoral candidate Somave Yosaee, from Larestan University of Medical Sciences, and colleagues found that zinc supplementation can lower the risk of mood disorders by an *impressive 28%*.

Supplement criteria: When choosing a zinc supplement, aim for a dosage between 7.5 and 15 mg. Many supplements offer around 30 mg, but that's usually more than you need. For better absorption, look for forms such as zinc picolinate, zinc bisglycinate or zinc citrate. I've found that zinc in the form of picolinate works best for me.

Directions for use: Take 7.5–15 mg of zinc most days of the week, noting that women usually need a bit less than men. Some studies suggest that taking zinc at night might improve sleep quality, so it can be a good idea to take it alongside your evening magnesium supplement.

6. Ginger

Ginger is packed with over *400 bioactive compounds* and boasts powerful anti-inflammatory and antioxidant properties. These can help with mental health issues related to inflammation in the body and brain. Ginger also supports serotonin and dopamine levels, which are key for mood regulation. Research by Dr Yu-Fang Lin from Zhejiang Hospital in China and colleagues showed that ginger not only helps relieve fatigue and depression but also improves sleep quality. A study out of Islamic Azad University led by Fatemeh Fadaki even found ginger extract to be an appropriate replacement for the potent pharmaceutical drug diazepam (Valium) in reducing anxiety symptoms.

Case study:

I started taking ginger around 2 years ago, and it transformed my health. Within a few weeks, I noticed increased energy levels and enhanced mental clarity. My sleep quality improved significantly, and I experienced better gut health, feeling less bloated and more comfortable overall. This simple addition to my diet led to a remarkable boost in my overall wellbeing, helping me feel more vibrant, focused, and balanced each day.

Supplement criteria: When choosing a ginger supplement, look for one that provides up to 1,200 mg of *Zingiber officinale*. Also, make sure it includes black pepper, which helps your body absorb the ginger better.

Directions for use: For best results, take 800–1,200 mg of ginger daily with your first meal and keep taking it consistently.

7. Vitamin C

You might think of vitamin C as just a remedy for colds, but it actually does a lot for your mental health. It helps manage stress and anxiety by regulating cortisol levels and has *antidepressant effects*.

For example, Dr Bettina Moritz from the Federal University of Santa Catarina and colleagues found that vitamin C supplementation can boost mood and reduce symptoms of depression and anxiety. This suggests that vitamin C could be a helpful addition to treating mood disorders.

Vitamin C is also essential for producing serotonin, dopamine, and norepinephrine—key neurotransmitters for mood regulation. Plus, it's a powerful antioxidant that protects your cells from damage and helps reduce inflammation, which can impact mental health.

Supplement criteria: When choosing a vitamin C supplement, aim for one that provides 500 mg of vitamin C. Liposomal vitamin C is a great option since it's known for higher absorption and may reach your bloodstream more effectively.

Directions for use: Take 500 mg of vitamin C daily. If you're dealing with active mental health symptoms, you can increase your dosage to 1,000 mg daily. Consistency is important—some research suggests you could see mood improvements in as little as 7 days. You don't need blood tests to start using vitamin C.

8. Curcumin

I've been taking curcumin daily for about 3 years, and the research by Dr Laura Fusar-Poli and her colleagues is a big reason why. Their study at the University of Catania reviewed 9 high-quality studies and found that curcumin is highly effective at reducing symptoms of depression and anxiety.

Curcumin is the main active ingredient in turmeric, the bright yellow spice. It's fantastic for fighting inflammation, managing cortisol levels, and acting as an antioxidant to protect your cells' energy-producing parts, called mitochondria.

Supplement criteria: When choosing a curcumin supplement, make sure it's **not just turmeric but specifically curcumin**, which is the active ingredient. Look for a supplement that's at least 90% curcumin—this will usually be highlighted on the label. If this information isn't listed, it's best to skip that product.

Also, pick a supplement that includes black pepper extract (*Piper nigrum*), as it can boost curcumin absorption **by up to 2,000%**. Aim for capsules containing 400–500 mg of curcumin.

Directions for use: Curcumin is generally safe for most people, but there is a rare risk of liver issues for some. To minimise this risk, start with a lower dose and watch for any side effects, such as yellowing of the skin, darker urine, nausea, unusual tiredness, weakness, or abdominal pain.

Here's a simple approach to start with curcumin:

- **Initial dose:** Begin with one 400–500 mg capsule every day for 3 months.
- **Monitor:** Get a liver function test after 3 months to check for any issues.

- **Adjust:** If all is well, you can increase to 800–1,000 mg once daily for another 3 months.

- **Follow-up:** After this period, have another liver function test to ensure everything is still okay.

If you experience no side effects and your doctor approves, you can continue with the higher dose. Expect to see benefits after 2–3 months of consistent use.

How do I maximise my targeted supplementation?

A good supplement plan can tackle some of the root causes of mental health issues and provide significant benefits. Just remember, supplements take time to work, so patience and consistency are key. Think of each one as a long-term boost to your mental wellbeing.

1. Get screened: Start by getting the recommended health screening tests listed earlier in this guide—especially for vitamin D, folate, vitamin B12, magnesium, zinc, and liver function. This will ensure your levels are safe and help you figure out what you need.

2. Consult your healthcare provider: Talk to your doctor or healthcare professional to make sure the supplements are right for you and won't interact with any medications you're taking.

3. Choose quality supplements: Stick to the supplement criteria mentioned for each one in this step. The quality, dosage, and form of the supplement matter for getting the best results.

4. Follow directions: Pay attention to when and how to take each supplement. Some work better at specific times of the day, so make sure you're following the instructions.

5. Set reminders: Use your phone to set reminders or place your supplements where you'll see them, like next to your coffee machine. This helps you remember to take them until it becomes a habit.

6. **Track your progress:** Keep notes on how you're feeling—changes in mood, energy, etc. This will help you see whether the supplements are making a difference.

7. **Adjust as needed:** Recheck your levels periodically to adjust dosages or stop supplements if necessary. This keeps your regimen safe and effective.

Step Two Checklist: Targeted Supplementation

You're now ready to dive into targeted supplementation for mental health. Use this checklist to help you get started and stay on track:

☐ **Understand the basics:** Make sure you've read and understood the targeted supplementation section. You should feel confident about how it can benefit your mental health.

☐ **Complete screening tests:** Finish all the recommended tests from the screening step to ensure the supplements are safe for you.

☐ **Consult your healthcare provider:** Go over your screening results and discuss the supplements you plan to use with your healthcare professional. They'll help you confirm that everything is safe and appropriate for you.

☐ **Choose the right supplements:** Buy only those supplements that meet the criteria outlined in this step. Look for therapeutic dosages and activated forms. Avoid ones with gluten, soy, alcohol, artificial flavours, and maltodextrin.

☐ **Prioritise your purchases:** If you can't buy all 8 supplements at once, start with the ones listed first in this step.

☐ **Set up reminders:** Make sure you have a reminder system in place to help you remember to take your supplements regularly.

☐ **Follow directions:** Start taking your supplements according to the directions provided for each one.

☐ **Move forward:** Once you've got this step down, move on to the sleep step.

Step Three: Sleep

In this sleep-focused step, we'll look at how refining your sleep routine can significantly enhance your mental wellbeing. We'll explore evidence-based strategies to help you improve your sleep, which is a crucial early step in boosting your mental health.

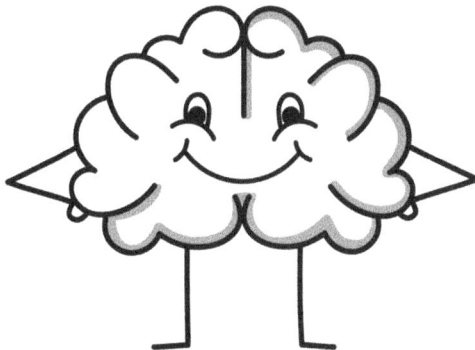

How's your sleep? According to a review of 22 studies by Dr Sophie Faulkner from the University of Manchester, about 80% of people with mental health challenges would answer this with "poor".

A major study by Dr Michael Wainberg and his team at the Centre for Addiction and Mental Health in Canada tracked nearly 90,000 people using accelerometers over a week. They found that people with mental health issues often experienced poorer sleep quality compared with the general population. The study showed a two-way relationship: *poor sleep can worsen mental health, and mental health struggles can lead to poor sleep*. Common issues included trouble falling asleep, staying asleep, or waking up too early.

Mental health symptoms such as fatigue, trouble concentrating, irritability, and low energy are often linked to poor sleep. Personally, I notice these symptoms when I haven't slept well, which highlights how much poor sleep can amplify mental health issues. Improving your sleep could help reduce these symptoms and boost overall mental wellbeing, yet it's often overlooked as a key factor in managing mental health.

How will sleep boost my mental health?

We know that adequate sleep is essential for good mental health, but what exactly is "adequate"? According to Dr Max Hirshkowitz and a panel of experts from Stanford University, as outlined by the National Sleep Foundation, aiming for *7 to 9 hours of uninterrupted sleep each night is ideal for supporting mental wellbeing.* Getting this amount of sleep can significantly benefit your mental health.

IMPROVED MOOD
Helps regulate emotions, boost positivity and reduce irritability, mood swings, sadness, and anxiety.

EMOTIONAL RESILIENCE
Sufficient sleep helps you manage and regulate your emotions more effectively.

STRESS REDUCTION
High quality sleep lowers stress levels and improves your ability to handle daily challenges by allowing your body to relax, recharge, and recover.

IMPROVED MENTAL HEALTH
Helps you manage mental health symptoms and improve treatment outcomes.

ENHANCED COGNITIVE FUNCTION
Improves attention, concentration and memory - making it easier to tackle complex tasks, solve problems, and make decisions.

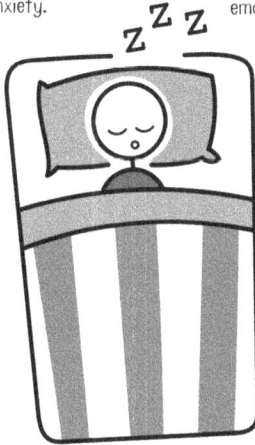

HORMONAL BALANCE
Helps regulate hormones, including stress (cortisol) and mood (serotonin and dopamine).

IMPROVED OVERALL WELLBEING
Quality sleep is essential for physical and mental health - supporting a strong immune system, high energy levels, and a positive outlook.

How do I improve my sleep?

Improving sleep hygiene can greatly enhance your sleep quality and quantity, but it takes time for your body to adjust. Be patient and consistent, and don't worry if you miss a step—just get back on track. Think of each new habit as a small investment that adds up over time. It may take some trial and error to find what works best for you, so focus on the strategies that fit your lifestyle and that you can maintain regularly.

1. Morning sun: Start your day by spending 15-30 minutes outside, exposing as much of your body and eyes to natural light as possible. Dr Nathaniel Watson, a sleep specialist, emphasises that morning sunlight is crucial for setting our circadian clock. I have been amazed at the difference this makes in my life.

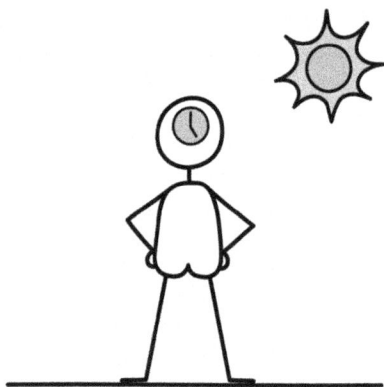

2. Consistent sleep schedule: Dr Colleen Lance recommends maintaining a regular sleep–wake schedule–going to bed and waking up at the same time every day, including weekends. Aim to get to sleep by 10 pm to help regulate your internal clock.

3. Restful sleep environment: Try to have noise levels below 35 dB, temperatures between 17 and 28 °C, and complete darkness. Use blackout curtains, earplugs, or sleep masks to block out disruptions. Dr Zachary Caddick from San Jose State Research Foundation has shown that these conditions are the best for good sleep.

4. Limit blue-light electronics before bed: Avoid screens for at least an hour before bed or use blue-light filters, and reduce screen brightness and increase screen colour warmness, as Harvard researchers found that blue light, emitted by phones, tablets, and computers, suppresses melatonin and disrupts sleep.

5. Avoid substances: Steer clear of nicotine, alcohol, caffeine, and excessive sugar within 4 hours of bedtime, as, according to Dr Christine Spadola from Florida Atlantic University, these substances can fragment sleep.

6. Invest in comfortable bedding: Think about those times you might have slept in a cheap budget motel with an uncomfortable mattress and pillows and recall the quality of your sleep. While you might think your bed at home does its job, think about what a mattress upgrade with new pillows might do to your sleep, in the same way that you might think of your current bed benefiting your sleep over one found in a budget motel. Invest in a comfortable and supportive mattress; after all, you spend one-third of your life lying on it. Find comfortable pillows and breathable bedding that suit your personal preferences.

7. Establish a relaxing bedtime routine: We all know routine in any facet of life promotes success and sleep is no different. Develop a pre-sleep routine to remind your body that it's time to prepare for sleep. This could include one of the other strategies in this list or other calming activities such as reading, taking a warm bath, practising relaxation techniques such as deep breathing or progressive muscle relaxation, or listening to soothing music. For me, it's a warm shower, magnesium supplement, and herbal tea with sleep-promoting ingredients.

8. Exercise regularly: Engage in physical activity on most days of the week, even if it is just an extended walk. Regular physical activity, especially *earlier in the day*, can significantly improve sleep quality, including for those with mental health challenges, as highlighted in Dr Oscar Lederman's 8-study meta-analysis.

9. Limit napping: Have you ever taken a nap that went a little longer than planned and then struggled to get to sleep that night? There's a reason for this. Napping lowers the body's accumulated need for sleep and disrupts circadian rhythm regulation. So, if you have difficulty falling asleep at night, limit daytime napping or keep it short (around 10–20 minutes), and avoid napping too close to bedtime.

What other sleeping aids can I use?

While the sleep hygiene habits mentioned should improve your sleep, some of you might still struggle. There are well-researched products that can enhance both the quality and quantity of your sleep. However, *before trying any of these, consult your doctor to ensure they're safe for you.* The products are listed in the order you should try them. Start with the first, and if that's not enough, continue using it while adding the next one on the list, and so forth. If you find that you need all these combined to get a good night's sleep, you might have a more serious sleep disorder and should see a sleep specialist.

1. Magnesium glycinate

I've been taking magnesium glycinate before bed for the past few years, and I have to say, my sleep has never been better. Dr Arman Arab from Isfahan University of Medical Sciences studied over 7,500 people and found solid evidence that magnesium helps with sleep. It's no surprise, really—this mineral is involved in over 300 chemical reactions in the body, many of which play a key role in regulating our sleep cycle.

Supplement criteria: The directions for using magnesium glycinate and the criteria for choosing the right supplement are already covered in the targeted supplementation section of this guide. But just to recap for sleep support—***stick to magnesium in the form of glycinate***.

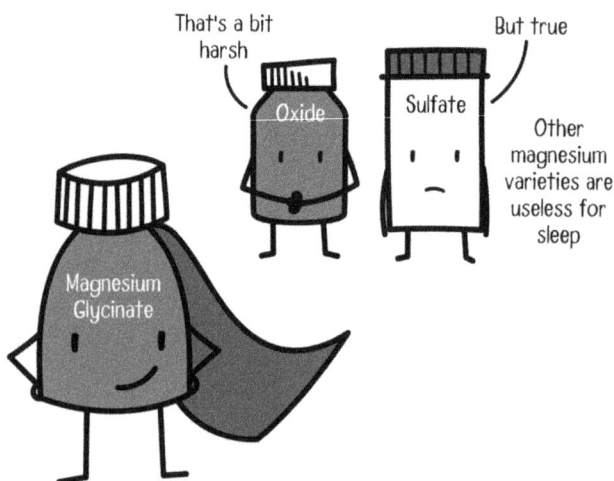

That's a bit harsh

Oxide

Sulfate

But true

Other magnesium varieties are useless for sleep

Magnesium Glycinate

Case study:

Georgia struggled for years to get a restful night's sleep, tossing and turning each night despite trying countless remedies. One day following a chat, I encouraged her to try magnesium glycinate and she decided to give it a go. To her amazement, after just a few nights, she began sleeping more soundly. Waking up refreshed became her new normal, and Georgia finally found the peaceful sleep she had been yearning for.

Directions for use: Take 200–300 mg of magnesium glycinate 30 to 60 minutes before bed.

2. Herbal tea (passionflower, chamomile, and lavender)

I've been enjoying herbal tea before bed for years, and my sleep is affected when I skip it. Professor Oliviero Bruni from Sapienza University found that herbal teas with ingredients including passionflower, chamomile, and lavender can really help with sleep. They work by interacting with GABA receptors in the brain, helping you feel more relaxed and calmer.

Supplement criteria: My tea has a mix of passionflower, chamomile, lavender, and an Aussie bush herb called jilungin (Terminalia canescens). I've tried a lot of different teas, but this combination works best for me. If you look for teas with passionflower, chamomile, and lavender, and want to be sure they're organic, I suggest using the same brand I do—Roogenic, which is made in Western Australia. It's been a game changer for my sleep quality!

Directions for use: Enjoy one tea bag about 60 to 90 minutes before bed. This gives you time for a bathroom trip before you settle in for the night.

3. Apigenin

Apigenin, found in certain herbs like chamomile, has sleep-inducing effects by activating the same GABA receptors in the brain as those targeted by anti-anxiety medications. A review by Daniel Kramer at Tally Health in New York highlights that apigenin stands out as a unique compound with significant influence on sleep.

Supplement criteria: Look for apigenin supplements in the range of 25–50 mg. It's best not to exceed 50 mg per day.

Directions for use: Take 25 mg of apigenin about 30 to 60 minutes before bed.

4. Theanine (L-theanine)

I've recently added L-theanine to my sleep routine once or twice a week after my busier days. L-theanine is great for promoting relaxation without making you drowsy. It boosts levels of calming neurotransmitters such as serotonin and GABA, which helps regulate sleep patterns and reduces stress and anxiety. Amanda Bulman, a doctoral candidate from the University of Canberra, and her colleagues reviewed 11 studies on L-theanine and found it effectively improves sleep quality on its own.

Supplement criteria: When looking for L-theanine supplements, aim for doses between 100–200 mg.

Directions for use: Take 100–200 mg of L-theanine 30–60 minutes before bed. Be aware that, for some people, it can cause vivid dreams or even sleepwalking. If you experience these side effects, stop using the supplement.

5. Myo-inositol

Dr Andrew Huberman, a neuroscientist and professor at Stanford University, has found that myo-inositol helps reset hormone signals that regulate sleep, leading to a more balanced and consistent sleep cycle.

Supplement criteria: Evidence suggests that a dose of 900 mg of myo-inositol may be effective for improving sleep patterns.

Directions for use: Take 900 mg if you wake up in the middle of the night and have trouble falling back asleep.

6. Glycine

Dr Janjira Soh from the National University Health System in Singapore reviewed research on glycine and found it particularly beneficial for the nervous system. One of the notable findings was that glycine administration can improve sleep.

Supplement criteria: Dose of 1–2 g.

Directions for use: Take 1–2 g of glycine 1 hour before bed. Use it up to 2–3 nights per week, but not every night.

7. Melatonin

Although I don't recommend using melatonin regularly, Fiona Auld and her team from the Department of Sleep Medicine in the UK reviewed 12 high-quality studies on melatonin. They found that melatonin can effectively reduce the time it takes to fall asleep and help regulate sleep–wake patterns, even for people with insomnia, compared with a placebo (a treatment that has no active ingredients). However, long-term, regular use disrupts your body's ability to produce its own melatonin, so to avoid this only take it irregularly.

Supplement criteria: Search for melatonin supplements that come in a 2 mg slow-release form.

Directions for use: Use melatonin only when needed, no more than 1 to 2 nights per week. Take it 30 minutes before bed.

Step Three Checklist: Sleep

You should now have a good grasp of how sleep affects your mental health and feel ready to boost your sleep habits and hygiene. Use this checklist to make sure you're on track with improving your sleep quality:

☐ **Understand sleep basics:** Get familiar with the basics of sleep by reading the sleep section.

☐ **Morning sunlight:** Try to get 15-30 minutes of direct natural light exposure on your skin and eyes right after you wake up. It helps set your internal clock.

☐ **Set a consistent sleep schedule:** Go to bed and wake up at similar times every day.

☐ **Comfortable sleep environment:** Make sure your bedroom is dark, quiet, and at a comfy temperature. This makes it easier to fall asleep.

☐ **Limit screen time:** Put away screens at least an hour before bed. The blue light can mess with your sleep.

☐ **Avoid stimulants and alcohol:** Stay away from caffeine, nicotine, sugar, and alcohol for at least 4 hours before bedtime.

☐ **Comfortable bedding:** Check that your mattress and pillows are comfortable and supportive. They play a big role in how well you sleep.

☐ **Relaxing bedtime routine:** Develop a soothing pre-sleep routine, such as enjoying a cup of herbal sleep tea, taking a warm bath, or reading a book.

☐ **Regular exercise:** Aim for regular exercise, ideally in the morning. It can help you sleep better.

☐ **Limit napping:** Keep naps short or avoid them if they mess with your night-time sleep.

☐ **Try sleep aids:** If you're still having trouble, experiment with different sleep aids one at a time to find what works best for you.

☐ **Consult a sleep specialist:** If you've tried everything and still have sleep issues, it might be time to see a sleep specialist.

☐ **Move on:** When you're ready, move on to the balanced nutrition part of the guide.

Step Four:
Balanced Nutrition

Our brains absorb between 20% and 40% of the nutrients and calories we consume. Let that sink in!

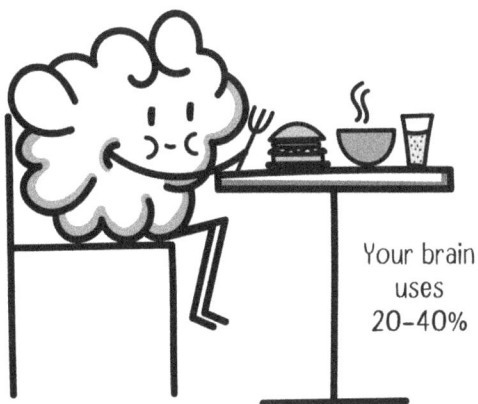

Your brain
uses
20-40%

Most people are not aware of this, and I think if they were, they might reconsider some of their nutritional choices. The foods we consume literally determine our brain health, and our brain health determines our mental health.

As recently as 2020, the Australian and New Zealand College of Psychiatrists updated their clinical practice guidelines for mood disorders, making specific recommendations around diet. This is such an important advancement!

The brain is also made up of 60% fat, and so if we are not consuming enough healthy fats, our brain will start relying on bad fats, resulting in all sorts of issues and mental health consequences.

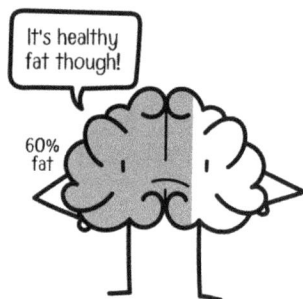

It's healthy fat though!

60% fat

In this step, we're going to explore how different foods can impact your mental health—both positively and negatively. We'll dive into mental health superfoods and how they can boost your wellbeing. Plus, I'll share some strategies to help you make the most of your diet for better mental health.

I'm really passionate about this topic! As a registered psychologist with a nutrition degree and a registered nutritionist in Australia, I've seen firsthand how important nutrition is for mental health.

It's crucial to rethink how we view food in relation to our mental wellbeing. Think of it as a simple choice: your food is either helping or hurting your mental health. Since your brain uses a lot of the nutrients you consume, making healthier choices can have a big impact. And don't forget about the "gut–brain connection"—I've mentioned it earlier in this guide, and it's a big factor too.

Dr Camille Lassale from University College, London, has examined 41 studies on how diet affects mental health, focusing on the benefits of a Mediterranean diet and the importance of avoiding pro-inflammatory foods. Her research suggests that these dietary habits can significantly protect mental health. This might also explain why people in blue zones—regions known for their long life spans—tend to have fewer mental health issues.

When you look online for foods that support mental health, it's easy to get overwhelmed by conflicting advice. This confusion often comes from hidden interests and sponsorships. To make things simpler, I've selected foods and nutrition tips based on solid, peer-reviewed research. My aim is to keep things straightforward and evidence-based, so you can focus on the foods that really support your mental wellbeing without getting bogged down by too many options.

How will balanced nutrition boost my mental health?

When it comes to food, we can make straightforward choices about whether what we eat will help or hurt our mental health. Different foods impact our mental wellbeing in various ways, either supporting or undermining it.

Neurotransmitters synthesis: Healthy food choices, rich in nutrients like tryptophan, boost neurotransmitters such as dopamine and serotonin, leading to more stable moods, according to research from Dr Arunkumar Dhailappan at Shri Nehru Maha Vidyalaya College of Arts and Science.

Anti-inflammatory: Eating anti-inflammatory foods can boost our mood and support brain health. Dr Edwin McDonald, a gastroenterologist, highlights how these foods help reduce inflammation in the body and contain beneficial compounds such as apigenin and luteolin, promoting overall wellbeing.

Antioxidant boost: Antioxidant-rich foods, such as those high in vitamins E and C, carotenoids, beta-carotene, flavonoids, and glutathione, are great for protecting brain cells and supporting mental health. These nutrients help combat oxidative stress (cell damage), which is linked to various mental health issues.

Enhanced gut health: Eating a balanced diet fosters a healthy gut microbiome and supports the gut–brain connection. A diverse range of beneficial bacteria from healthy foods boosts neurotransmitter production, enhances immunity, and improves digestion. These balanced gut bacteria also help maintain 95% of our serotonin, which is vital for mood regulation.

Balance hormones: Balanced nutrition can positively influence hormone levels, including those involved in stress response and mood regulation. Eating the right foods supports hormone function, promoting a balanced mood and overall wellbeing.

Nutrient supply: Whole foods provide essential nutrients such as vitamins, minerals, omega-3 fatty acids, and electrolytes, which are crucial for brain health. These nutrients support brain function, energy production, and neurotransmitter synthesis. In contrast, processed foods often lack these vital nutrients. Our brains are also made up of 60% fat and consist of large amounts of vitamins and minerals, so we need an adequate supply to allow our brains to function well.

Blood sugar regulation: Maintaining stable blood sugar levels is achieved through good nutrition, which helps ensure steady energy and a positive mood, and prevents the fatigue often associated with fluctuating blood sugar.

Hydration: Fresh and healthy foods are hydrating, which supports neurotransmitter production and helps supply our brains with fresh oxygen and nutrients. Processed foods can lead to dehydration and negatively impact mental health—think alcohol and hangovers!

Better pH balance: Nutritious foods help maintain a balanced pH in the body, which supports overall health and brain function. Processed foods can disrupt this balance.

Energy boost: Whole, fresh foods provide sustained energy and mental clarity, helping to combat fatigue and irritability. Unlike processed foods that cause energy spikes and crashes, healthy foods offer a steady source of energy, supporting better mental health.

Increased neuroplasticity: Certain nutrients from whole foods support neuroplasticity (the brain's ability to adapt and reorganise). This is crucial for stress response and emotional regulation. Opting for nutritious foods helps enhance neuroplasticity, benefiting mental health.

Brain oxygen and blood: Foods that promote good blood flow and oxygen delivery to the brain support optimal mental health. Healthy nutrition enhances our blood vessel function, ensuring our brains receive the oxygen and nutrients they need to thrive.

Reduced stress: Eating a balanced diet helps our bodies handle stress better, which can make a big difference in our mental health. On the flip side, processed foods can make stress and mood issues worse, so sticking to healthier options can support a calmer, more resilient mindset.

Stronger immune system: Our immune systems play a key role in our mental wellbeing. Nutritious foods keep our immune systems strong, which can help us stay healthy and feel better mentally. A well-rounded diet is like giving our immune system a boost, leading to better overall mental health.

Better sleep: Nutritious foods typically contain sleep-promoting nutrients (e.g. tryptophan and magnesium), while innutritious foods not only lack these nutrients, but also contain other additives that are known sleep disruptors (e.g. processed sugar and caffeine).

What nutritional choices are good for my mental health?

Let's dive into the foods that can truly boost your mental health. I've ranked them based on how beneficial they are, so the top ones are the most effective. You don't need to love every single food on the list—just pick the ones you enjoy and try to add more of them to your diet. The goal isn't to eat everything mentioned, but to increase your intake of foods that can support your mental wellbeing. I've also highlighted a special group of mental health superfoods, making it easier for you to spot the best options for your brain.

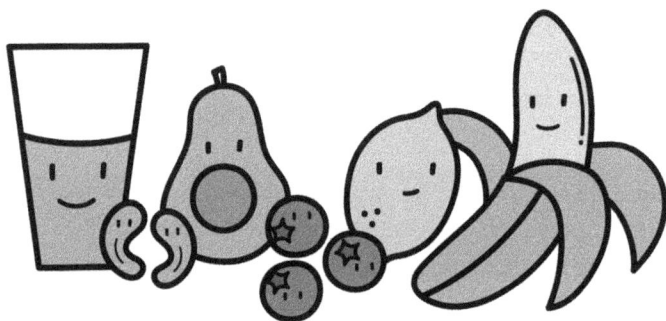

MENTAL HEALTH SUPERFOODS

1. Mental health superfoods

Mental health superfoods are the cream of the crop when it comes to nutrient-packed foods. They're loaded with vitamins, minerals, antioxidants, and other compounds that are proven to support brain and mental health. While some of these super-foods might overlap with other food categories, this list focuses on the ones you should prioritise.

Ideally, try to include at least one of these superfoods in your diet every day. If you're dealing with mental health challenges, add one to each meal. These superfoods can really make a difference in supporting your mental wellbeing.

Prioritise these:

- organic celery juice (fresh)
- organic spirulina
- wild blueberries
- broccoli sprouts (young broccoli plant sprouts)
- wild-caught salmon
- natural and raw cashews and walnuts
- pumpkin and chia seeds
- lemons
- avocados
- bananas

Case study:

James was struggling with mental health issues, including panic attacks and depression. After discussing his diet, we found he was consuming too much sugar and trans fats (see the pages that follow for more on these). We identified superfoods he liked, such as avocados, wild blueberries, cashews, walnuts, and fish, and incorporated them into his diet. Within a month of these changes, James noticed tangible improvements in his mental health, highlighting the powerful impact of balancing diet by making small adjustments.

2. Greens

Go green with your diet! Professor Dominika Głąbska from Warsaw University of Life Sciences reviewed 61 studies on the relationship between vegetables and mental health and found green vegetables can boost optimism and self-confidence while also reducing psychological distress and protecting against mental health issues.

Among these greens, celery juice really stands out. It's been used as medicine in the Eastern world for thousands of years, and now research supports its benefits. Dr Gasem Abu-Taweel from Jazan University found that celery has strong effects on biochemical disorders, including those related to mental health. Celery juice is an excellent hydration tonic, packed with vitamins, minerals, antioxidants, and mineral salts that help calm the brain and nervous system. Plus, it contains luteolin, which supports neurotransmitter production linked to mental wellbeing.

For the best results, drink freshly juiced celery juice first thing in the morning on an empty stomach—no need to dilute it with water.

Prioritise these:

- celery juice
- coriander
- broccoli
- asparagus
- spinach
- beans
- barley grass juice powder
- spirulina
- other herbs: mint, basil, thyme, rosemary, parsley, oregano

3. Berries

All berries are great for your mental health, and the darker the berry, the better. Wild blueberries, in particular, stand out. These small, naturally growing berries—found mostly in North America—contain 33% more anthocyanins and twice the antioxidants of regular blueberries. Research by Jeni Fisk from the University of Reading found that 4 weeks of daily wild blueberry consumption significantly reduced mental health symptoms compared to a placebo (fake berries).

Frozen wild blueberries are just as nutritious, if not more so, than fresh ones. While they might not be in your local super-market, you can usually find them in the frozen section of a good health food store. They're smaller than regular blueberries, so aim to consume one-half to one cup daily.

Prioritise these:

- wild blueberries
- blueberries
- blackberries
- raspberries
- strawberries
- cranberries
- goji berries
- elderberries
- boysenberries
- mulberries

4. Oily fish and shellfish

In blue zones—regions where people live longer and have lower rates of chronic diseases—fish is a dietary staple. While fish alone isn't the only factor behind their impressive longevity and mental health, it certainly plays a role. A study by Yeonji Yang from Korea's Kyung Hee University involving 109,764 participants found strong evidence that fish consumption benefits mental health.

Among all fish, salmon and oysters are top choices for mental health. Aim to include them in your diet 2 to 3 times a week, along with fish oil supplements for added benefit.

Prioritise these:

- wild-caught salmon
- sardines
- rainbow trout

- herring
- anchovies
- Atlantic mackerel
- Pacific halibut
- pollock
- oysters
- mussels
- clams

5. Nuts and seeds

Dr Andrew Saul, a therapeutic nutritionist and editor-in-chief of Orthomolecular Medicine News Service, once mentioned that "several handfuls of cashews provide 1,000–2,000 mg of tryptophan, which will work as well as prescription antidepressants." While I don't fully agree with the comparison to antidepressants, he's right about cashews being rich in tryptophan, a key component in serotonin production—the same neurotransmitter that many antidepressants target.

Dr Rubén Fernández-Rodríguez from Universidad de Castilla-La Mancha also found, in his review of 66,418 people, that higher nut consumption is linked to a lower risk of depression and better mood.

When it comes to nuts and seeds, cashews and walnuts stand out for mental health. Walnuts, which interestingly resemble a brain, not only boost mental wellbeing but, according to research from Mauritz Herselman at the University of South Australia, also improve mental health markers and reduce stress-related changes in metabolism and gut microbiota. For optimal benefits, consume raw, unsalted nuts—about one-third of a cup of walnuts and one-third of a cup of cashews daily.

Prioritise these:

- walnuts

- almonds
- cashews
- Brazil nuts
- pistachios
- hazelnuts
- pecans
- macadamia nuts
- pumpkin seeds
- chia seeds

6. Fruit and vegetables

Researcher Neel Ocean from the University of Leeds analysed 7 years of data and found that adding just one more portion of fruits and vegetables to your daily diet can boost mental wellbeing as much as 8 days of 10-minute walks. Plus, eating an extra 100g of fruits and veggies can lower your risk of depression by 3%–5%, according to a review of 27 studies by Faezeh Saghafian from Tehran University of Medical Sciences.

A study involving 4,241 participants led by Putu Novi Arfirsta Dharmayani from Macquarie University also shows that consuming at least 4 servings of fruit and 5 servings of vegetables a day can lead to a 19% and 25% lower risk of developing depression, respectively, over 15 years compared with those eating one serving or less.

I know berries and greens are fruit and vegetables and could therefore sit within this section; however, due to their superiority in assisting mental health functions, they rightly deserve their own categories earlier in this section. Any fresh or frozen fruits and vegetables will benefit your mental health. Lemons and avocados are 2 superior examples—consider squeezing one whole lemon in a glass with water upon waking in the morning and aim for 3 to 5 avocados per week.

Prioritise these:

- lemons
- oranges
- bananas
- avocados
- kale
- bell peppers (capsicums)
- pineapple
- sweet potatoes

What nutritional choices are bad for my mental health?

When it comes to nutrition, we can think of our choices as either helping or hurting our mental health. To make things easier, I've categorised harmful nutritional groups for you, mostly focusing on ultra-processed foods. These groups are listed in order of how damaging they can be to mental health, with the most harmful first.

While it's not realistic to expect you'll completely eliminate these from your life, being aware of them can help you make better choices, especially during tough times. It takes about 60 days to build a new habit or break an old one, so don't be too hard on yourself if you slip up occasionally. It's all part of the process.

1. Alcohol

Unfortunately for those of us who enjoy a drink, alcohol is harmful for our mental health. Research by Professor Katherine Keyes from Columbia University, which looked at 57,276 older adults across 19 countries, shows that alcohol consumption can directly lead to mental health issues. In other words, drinking alcohol independently increases the risk of experiencing mental health problems.

Avoid these:

- beer
- spirits
- cocktails
- white wine
- liqueurs

2. Processed sugar

Many of us know that processed sugar is bad for physical health, but it's also a culprit for mental health issues. Dr Angela Jacques from Queensland University of Technology reviewed over 300 studies and found that high-processed-sugar diets are linked to cognitive problems such as impaired brain plasticity, as well as increased anxiety and depression.

Avoid these:

- dextrose
- corn syrup
- sucrose
- fructose
- table sugar
- soft drinks, energy drinks and sports drinks
- fruit juices with added sugars
- breakfast cereals
- doughnuts
- candies
- chocolate and ice cream
- packaged desserts
- ketchup and barbecue sauce
- sweetened coffee drinks

3. Trans fats

Eating too many trans fats can nearly double your risk of depression. This finding comes from a 6-year study with over 12,000 participants led by Professor Almudena Sánchez-Villegas from the University of Las Palmas de Gran Canaria.

This research has been enough to motivate me to cut down on trans fats significantly.

Avoid these:

- commercial baked goods (such as cakes, cookies and pies)
- microwave popcorn
- frozen pizza
- refrigerated dough (such as biscuits and rolls)
- fried foods (including French fries, doughnuts and fried chicken)
- partially hydrogenated vegetable oils

4. Food additives (artificial colours, sweeteners, flavourings, and preservatives)

Food additives are used to enhance taste, freshness, or appearance, but they can impact mental health negatively. Ruo-Gu Xiong from Sun Yat-sen University found that these additives can contribute to anxiety, depression, and other mental health issues. Since some additives are hidden in ingredient lists, it's important to read labels carefully.

Avoid these:

- artificial food colouring (tartrazine, Allura Red, red 40, yellow 5)
- artificial sweeteners (aspartame, saccharin, sucralose)
- monosodium glutamate (MSG)
- high-fructose corn syrup (HFCS)
- sodium benzoate

- butylated hydroxyanisole (BHA)
- butylated hydroxytoluene (BHT)
- nitrites and nitrates
- artificial flavourings

5. Industrial and processed seed oils

Dr Uma Naidoo, a nutritional psychiatrist at Harvard Medical School, advises that the number one food group to avoid for brain health is industrial and processed seed oils, which are high in omega-6 fatty acids. Unlike the beneficial omega-3s in fish, omega-6s can increase inflammation in the body and brain. For better brain health, opt for healthier oils such as olive and avocado oil instead.

Avoid these:

- soybean oil
- corn oil
- rapeseed (the source of canola oil)
- cottonseed oil
- sunflower oil
- safflower seeds

6. Sodium

You've probably noticed the pattern: what's bad for our physical health can also harm our mental health, and processed salt is no exception. Research by Celeste Ferraris from the University of Newcastle found that high sodium intake is linked to increased depression, anxiety, and stress. While you don't need to cut out all salt, it's important to be mindful of overconsuming processed salty foods.

Avoid these:

- processed meats (such as bacon, sausage, and deli meats)
- canned soups

- potato chips and other salty snacks
- condiments (such as soy, tomato, and barbecue sauces)
- cheese, particularly processed cheeses
- instant noodles and ramen
- frozen dinners and prepackaged meals
- fast food (such as burgers, fries, and chicken nuggets)
- salted butter and margarine
- pizza
- bread and rolls
- breakfast cereals

7. Saturated fats

When it comes to fats, we have 2 friends and 2 foes. Saturated fats are our second foe, though they're less damaging than trans fats. Han Chen from Hangzhou Normal University found that diets high in saturated fats, such as those in butter and cheese, were linked to higher risks of depression and anxiety among 126,819 people in the UK. You don't need to cut out saturated fats entirely, but it's wise to be mindful of consuming too much. I certainly continue my love of cheese.

Avoid these:

- butter and lard
- cheese (such as cheddar and feta)
- cream
- ice cream
- pork belly
- lamb chops
- chicken skin
- processed meats (such as sausages, bacon, and salami)
- beef burgers
- processed snack foods (such as chips and crackers)
- fried foods (such as French fries and fried chicken)

- baked goods made with butter, lard, or palm oil (such as cakes, cookies, and pastries)

8. Caffeine

I'll start by saying I love coffee and don't discourage you from using it if it works for you—there are even studies showing it benefits depression. However, if you're prone to anxiety, you might want to watch your caffeine intake. While some people handle caffeine just fine, it can trigger anxiety and panic attacks in others. A review of 10 studies by Lisa Klevebrant from Uppsala University found that caffeine significantly increased panic attacks in people with an anxiety disorder and heightened anxiety in both those with and without the disorder. Caffeine can make you feel more anxious by affecting relaxation, increasing heart rate, and disrupting sleep. It's not just in coffee —caffeine is also found in many other foods and drinks.

Avoid these:

- coffee
- tea (black, green, white, oolong)
- most energy drinks
- some soft drinks (Coke, Pepsi, Mountain Dew)
- chocolate
- some energy bars and gels
- some over-the-counter and prescription medications, such as pain relievers, cold remedies, and weight loss pills

How do I optimise my nutrition?

Optimising our diet is key for our mental health. Food preferences are unique to each person, and what works best for one person may be different from what works for others. While we can occasionally enjoy less healthy options, it's important to focus on beneficial nutrition as often as possible. Here are some practical strategies to enhance your nutritional habits:

1. Know your foods: Learn which foods are beneficial and which are harmful. This helps you make better choices and avoid confusion from misleading nutrition information and advertising.

2. Evaluate your diet: Look at your current eating habits. Use a food journal or nutrition app to track what you consume and spot areas for improvement.

3. Identify challenges: Recognise what's holding you back from better nutrition. A review of 15 studies by Dr Heather Colquhoun at the University of Toronto shows that identifying these barriers is crucial to making lasting changes. Find solutions to overcome them.

4. Smart shopping: When grocery shopping, focus on buying beneficial foods and limit harmful ones. This way, you'll have healthier options at home.

5. Plan your meals: Create a weekly menu that includes plenty of nutritious foods and minimises harmful ones. This could be as simple as ensuring breakfast each morning is packed with beneficial nutrients or ensuring dinner contains beneficial nutrients. For me, I like to ensure my breakfast is ultra healthy. I start with freshly squeezed lemon water and usually have a water-based smoothie packed with superfoods or pot-set natural yoghurt with cashews, walnuts, pumpkin seeds, chia seeds, and berries.

6. Start small: Begin with manageable changes. For instance, try adding one superfood and cutting out one unhealthy food each day, then gradually expand to doing this in more meals.

7. Diversify your diet: Incorporate a variety of nutrients from different beneficial food groups, with an emphasis on superfoods.

8. Try new foods: Break out of your usual food routine by sampling new and different foods. This can help you discover healthy options you might enjoy.

Step Four Checklist: Balanced Nutrition

You should now have a solid understanding of how balanced nutrition impacts your mental health and feel ready to use strategies to improve your diet. Use this checklist to guide your efforts and ensure you're making the most of this step:

☐ **Nutrition content concepts:** Review the nutrition section to make sure you grasp the key concepts.

☐ **Know your nutrition:** Be familiar with both beneficial and harmful foods for mental health.

☐ **Evaluate your diet:** Evaluate your current diet to identify areas for improvement and recognise any barriers.

☐ **Improve food access:** Ensure your home is stocked with more beneficial foods and fewer harmful ones. Consider reorganising your pantry and updating your shopping list.

☐ **Incorporate superfoods:** Consume at least 1 superfood every day and ideally 3.

☐ **Boost beneficial foods:** Boost your intake of foods that support mental wellbeing.

☐ **Reduce harmful foods:** Cut back on foods that negatively impact your mental health.

☐ **Move forward:** Move on to the movement step of this guide.

Step Five: Movement

In this movement-focused step, we'll explore how physical activity impacts mental health and how you can optimise your movement routine based on the latest research. When we look at different forms of exercise and physical activity, we can categorise them all as movement. The goal is to integrate more movement into your life, recognising that *any activity involving muscle contraction is our goal*.

Although we know movement positively affects mental health, fitting regular exercise into our busy lives can be challenging due to time constraints and fluctuating motivation. Research from the University of Oxford by Sammi Chekroud involving 1.2 million people found that those who exercise experience *43 more days of improved mental health each year* compared with those who don't exercise.

Academics including Dr Cristy Phillips from Arkansas State University have found evidence for why this might be the case. *Movement that causes your muscles to contract secretes chemicals including myokines* directly into your bloodstream. *Myokines are small proteins that travel to our brains and act as antidepressants.* Because of this some scientists have referred to these myokines as "hope" molecules. These hope molecules have also been shown to cross the blood–brain barrier, meaning they will go directly to your brain and positively impact your mental health.

Dr Andreas Heissel reviewed over 40 studies and found that exercise has such a strong effect on reducing mental health symptoms that it should be considered a standard mental health treatment option.

Beyond myokines, which are directly linked to exercise, movement also boosts neurotransmitters such as dopamine and serotonin. These neurotransmitters further enhance your mood and mental wellbeing.

How will movement boost my mental health?

When you think of physical activity and exercise, do you think you must break a sweat for it to count? It's not the case! That's why we talk about *movement* instead of just *exercise*. Any kind of movement that gets our muscles working can release myokines, which act like natural antidepressants and cross the blood–brain barrier to boost our mood. So, even if you're not doing intense workouts, adding regular movement to your routine—like taking a brisk walk or stretching—can make a big difference in how you feel.

Increase in myokines: When we move, our muscles release myokines, often called "hope" molecules. These act like natural antidepressants and can boost our mood. So, if you're not moving, you're missing out on these free mood enhancers!

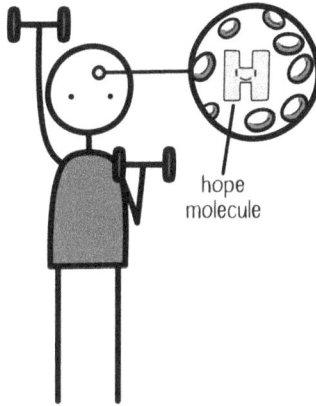

hope
molecule

Endorphins boost: These brain hormones block pain and make us feel good. Research by Kathleen Mikkelsen shows that exercise ramps up endorphin levels, giving us a natural high.

Enhanced neurotransmitter regulation: Aerobic exercise helps balance neurotransmitters such as serotonin and dopamine, which are crucial for mental health. Saskia Heijnen's research highlights how movement supports these brain chemicals.

Stress reduction: Exercise lowers stress hormones such as cortisol and helps us handle stress better. Even 20–30 minutes of cardio can cut down on stress and give you a distracting break from negative thoughts, as found by Professor Erica Jackson.

Improved sleep: Just 30 minutes of daily movement can enhance both the quality and duration of our sleep. Majd Alnawwar's review of 23 studies shows that regular exercise can add up to 15 minutes of extra sleep compared with a sedentary lifestyle.

Increased blood flow: Moving around boosts blood flow, which means our brains get more oxygen and nutrients. This helps our brains stay healthy and supports our mental wellbeing.

Social interaction: Exercising in groups can improve our social connections and sense of community. This social connectedness is crucial for mental health, as we'll explore further in the social engagement section of this guide.

Reduction of inflammation: Movement helps lower inflammation, which is linked to mental health issues. Dr Kent Langston's research from Harvard Medical School found that exercise activates immune cells that fight inflammation.

Improved self-esteem: Just being active can boost our self-esteem and self-worth, according to an analysis of 38 studies out of Central South University led by Dr Mingli Liu.

Brain structure: Movement promotes the growth of new neurons and improves brain plasticity. This helps us adapt to new experiences and handle mental health challenges better.

What movement types are there?

Finding movement types you enjoy and can stick with is key to boosting your mental health. It's not about doing intense workouts or forcing yourself into a strict routine. The goal is to explore different types of movement and see what fits best into your life. Remember, any movement that gets your muscles working releases those hope molecules, giving you a natural mental health boost.

The US National Institute on Aging suggests trying out different categories of activities to cover all the bases for your mental wellbeing. By mixing things up and incorporating movement from each category, you'll get the most well-rounded benefits for your mind and body. The idea is to experiment until you find what makes you feel good and can become a regular part of your routine.

ENDURANCE/AEROBIC	STRENGTH OR RESISTANCE
Involves continuous, rhythmic activity that's kept at a moderate to high intensity over an extended period.	Uses resistance to muscular contractions to build strength, increase anaerobic endurance, and enhance the size of skeletal muscles. Also called weight training.

ENDURANCE/AEROBIC

Involves continuous, rhythmic activity that's kept at a moderate to high intensity over an extended period.

- walking
- running
- cycling
- swimming
- dancing
- gardening
- housework
- sports (tennis, football, basketball etc.)

STRENGTH OR RESISTANCE

Uses resistance to muscular contractions to build strength, increase anaerobic endurance, and enhance the size of skeletal muscles. Also called weight training.

- weightlifting
- resistance band exercises
- push ups, sit ups, planks etc.
- climbing stairs
- carrying things (groceries, laundry, children etc.)

FLEXIBILITY AND MOBILITY

Involves moving your joints through their full range of motion, which helps improve their stability and flexibility.

- yoga
- pilates
- bending down, reaching up and stretching in regular movement like: picking up a child, grabbing items up high or down low, tying your shoes etc.

BALANCE AND STABILITY

Focuses on strengthening the muscles that help keep you upright, such as your legs and core.

- tai chi
- walking backward
- balance exercises on unstable surfaces
- using a wobble or balance board
- walking heel-to-toe in a straight line
- walking with a weighted backpack

Case study:

Maria was dealing with anxiety and low energy levels. I asked about her daily routine and realised she wasn't getting much exercise. We decided to start small by adding a daily walk to her schedule, right after her morning coffee. This simple change made it easy to remember and stick to. Within a few weeks, Maria noticed she had more energy, felt less anxious, and her overall mood improved significantly.

How do I increase my movement?

Every bit of movement you add acts like a small dose of antidepressant for your brain. Start slowly and stay persistent— as remember that forming a new habit usually takes around 60 days. I've listed strategies in order of importance to help you prioritise. Not every strategy will fit perfectly, so keep experimenting until you find what makes it easier for you to fit movement into your routine.

1. Explore different activities: Experiment with various forms of movement to discover what you enjoy most. Research led by Wenjing Yan from Beijing Sport University shows that enjoying the activity is key to maintaining long-term engagement. Essentially, finding pleasure in movement is more important than being highly skilled at it for staying motivated.

2. Plan your schedule: According to Dr Erin Hoare from the Baker Heart and Diabetes Institute, the biggest barriers to movement are time constraints and fatigue. Think about your typical weekly schedule, noting when you usually have free time and when you feel most energised. Use these insights to carve out time for movement, treating it as a non-negotiable appointment with yourself. For me, it's immediately after work.

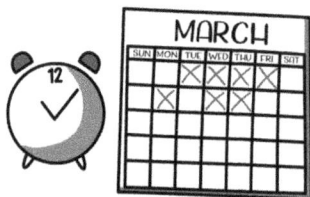

3. Integrate movement into daily life: Find simple ways to be more active in your daily routine. Walk to a coffee shop that's a bit further away, cycle to work, take the stairs instead of the lift, or do household chores manually. These small adjustments can significantly increase muscle contractions, providing more antidepressant effects for your brain. I apply this one in my life every day!

4. Monitor your progress: Use a fitness tracker or a journal to keep tabs on your movement habits. A study involving 7,454 people led by Dr Liliana Laranjo from the University of Sydney found that people who track their activity levels are more likely to stay active.

5. Set reminders: Use your phone or calendar to set reminders for your planned movement sessions. Research analysing 55 studies by Dr Daniel Collado-Mateo from Rey Juan Carlos University shows that reminders can boost your likelihood of following through.

6. Start small and build up: A review of 48 studies by Dr Gro Samdal from the University of Bergen emphasises the importance of starting with small, manageable movement goals and gradually increasing them. Begin with short, easy movement sessions and slowly ramp up both the duration and intensity to more easily reach your goal.

7. Make it social: Try working out with a friend, joining a group class, or participating in team sports to boost your motivation and accountability. A study led by Gabrielle Lindsay Smith from Victoria University, which reviewed findings from 27 studies, found that social support increases physical activity.

8. Keep it varied: Mix up your routine with different types of movement, such as cardio, strength training, flexibility exercises, and balance work. This not only keeps things interesting but also ensures you're targeting different muscle groups, allowing you to continue moving even if one part of your body is sore.

Step Five Checklist: Movement

You should now have a clear understanding of how movement affects mental health and feel ready to put strategies into practice. This checklist is designed to help you boost your overall movement and enhance your mental wellbeing:

☐ **Understand movement:** Review the movement step and make sure you grasp the key concepts.

☐ **Explore activities:** Try various different forms of movement to discover which ones you enjoy most and feel are best for you.

☐ **Plan your schedule:** Allocate specific times in your week when you're most energised and have free time for movement.

☐ **Integrate daily movement:** Look for opportunities to add movement into your daily routine, such as taking the stairs instead of the lift.

☐ **Track your progress:** Keep a record of your movement activities and achievements.

☐ **Set reminders:** Use alarms or calendar alerts to remind you of your planned movement sessions.

☐ **Start small:** Begin with manageable movement goals and gradually increase them.

☐ **Make it social:** Engage in movement activities with others to boost motivation and enjoyment.

☐ **Diversify activities:** Include a variety of movement types in your routine to maximise benefits.

☐ **Increase movement:** Ensure you're moving more than before and progressing from your initial levels.

☐ **Move to the next step:** Once you've established your movement routine, proceed to the social engagement step.

Step Six:
Social Engagement

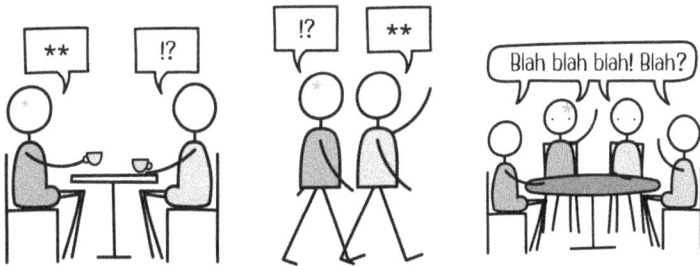

Connecting with others and having strong relationships are some of the most important factors for both our mental and physical health. Your social wellbeing is all about how you interact and build connections with people in your life. This includes the quality of your relationships, the support you get from your social network, and how engaged and fulfilled you feel in your social interactions.

In this step, we'll explore how being socially connected impacts mental health, look at some statistics on social connection, and share some easy, practical tips to help you boost your social wellbeing.

Dr Julianne Holt-Lunstad, Professor of Psychology and Neuroscience at Brigham Young University, led a review of 34 years of research highlighting the incredible benefits of staying socially connected. Her studies show that maintaining strong social connections can be as beneficial for your health as avoiding smoking or heavy drinking. In fact, her research suggests that staying socially engaged is ***twice as effective*** at boosting physical and mental health as maintaining a healthy weight.

In 2020, the World Health Organization noted an increase in mental health challenges around the globe, influenced by the COVID-19 pandemic. The pandemic underscored how much happier we all are when we can see our friends and family and interact with people in our communities. It revealed how crucial social connections are for our wellbeing, revealing areas where we can grow and improve our support systems. This experience highlights the need for us to strengthen our connections and find new ways to support each other, enhancing mental health for everyone.

How will social engagement boost my mental health?

Humans are naturally social beings, and our relationships are vital for our emotional wellbeing. Prioritising social connections is essential for maintaining good mental health. Engaging in social activities, fostering positive relationships, and reaching out for support when needed can enhance our mental health in many ways.

Better mental health: Having a strong social network can make a big difference. A review of 24 studies by Jingyi Wang from University College London shows that good social support leads to better treatment outcomes and fewer relapses. Additionally, Mengyun Luo from the University of Sydney studied 33,338 people and found staying socially active is linked to fewer mental health challenges overall.

Connectedness: Social connections help fight loneliness by creating a sense of belonging. Professor Manfred Beutel from Johannes Gutenberg University led a study of over 15,000 people that found connection is a serious health protector. It's linked to higher experiences of wellbeing, happiness, calmness, and healthy behaviours and less frequent doctor visits.

Improved cognition: Social engagement helps keep our brains sharp by involving activities that need us to use our attention, memory, and problem-solving skills. Dr Elvira Lara from Universidad Autónoma de Madrid found that feeling socially connected and engaged can lead to an increase in cognitive function over time, while Professor Ming Wen from the University of Utah showed that just staying socially active can improve cognitive health.

Reduced stress: Dr Daniel Campagne's research, analysing 42 studies, revealed that maintaining social connections helps manage stress and lower levels of stress hormones such as cortisol. This aligns with findings from the Centers for Disease Control and Prevention in the USA, which highlight the positive effects of socialising on reducing stress.

Healthier behaviours: The Centers for Disease Control and Prevention found that when people have strong, supportive relationships, they're more likely to make healthier choices, such as exercising regularly, getting enough sleep, and avoiding substance misuse. Basically, having a solid social network can really help you with sticking to good habits and overall wellness.

Long-term health benefits: Dr Julianne Holt-Lunstad's research including over 300,000 people found that having strong social relationships can boost your chances of living longer by 50%! This highlights how valuable good social connections are for your overall health and wellbeing. So, staying connected with others is a great way to support your longevity and happiness.

Improved mood: Jessica Martino from Tufts University School of Nutrition Research found that our social connections really impact our mood. Spending time with others often brings laughter, enjoyment, and positive experiences. These interactions can boost our mood and lead to greater happiness and contentment.

Emotional support: Social interactions give us a way to express our emotions and get support. Talking about our feelings, thoughts, and concerns with others can offer comfort, lower stress, and boost emotional wellbeing. Social networks also let us learn from others and share coping strategies, which helps build resilience and problem-solving skills. Connecting with people who face similar challenges can provide validation and understanding, making us feel less isolated.

Increased self-esteem: Positive social interactions with others enhance self-esteem according to a study by Dr Wing-Yee Cheung from the University of Southampton.

Reduction in rumination: Getting involved with others can be a great way to shift your focus away from negative thoughts and worries. It's kind of like a form of mindfulness—when you're chatting and spending time with people, you're more likely to be present and enjoying those positive interactions.

Case study:

I'm a social person and after the isolation of COVID-19, like many, I noticed I was less enthusiastic, and I felt somewhat disconnected. I realised I needed to re-engage socially, so I reached out to friends, scheduled regular get-togethers and made the most of face-to-face interactions. I also decided to try something new—group Pilates classes. I noticed an immediate benefit; I felt more connected, happier, and energised, which showed me the importance of social engagement for my mental wellbeing.

How do I enhance my social engagement?

Finding time for social activities can be a challenge, but the benefits for our wellbeing are definitely worth it. Staying connected with others has a big impact on our overall health and happiness.

Remember, it's perfectly fine if not all suggestions work for you immediately. The key is to stay open to new ideas and allow yourself to explore what feels right and works best. Habits take time to form, so be patient with yourself. Here are some positive strategies to help you get started:

1. Build on previous steps: If socialising feels tough, it's okay. Hopefully, you've already made some progress with earlier steps in this guide to build up your confidence for social interactions.

2. Start small: Think of social activities as a series of small steps. Begin with things that you're comfortable with and that match your interests and current mental health.

3. Enjoy everyday interactions: Simple things, such as chatting with the cashier at the shop or asking your barista how their day is going, can boost your sense of connection and belonging, according to the research findings of Dr Gillian Sandstrom from the University of British Columbia.

4. Face-to-face matters: Face-to-face interactions are better for your mental health compared with digital chats, according to a study by Dr Stefan Stieger. So, while keeping in touch online is still valuable, try to prioritise in-person meet-ups when you can.

5. Host gatherings: Invite friends or family over for a casual get-together, such as a movie night or potluck dinner. Hosting can help you build stronger connections and make it harder to back out.

6. Try new activities: Get involved in new activities that interest you, such as joining a social club, volunteering, educational or recreational activities, or attending classes. Any new engagement adds to your social life and can help you feel more connected. For me, it's been group Pilates classes.

7. Plan your social time: Time and energy are commonly cited as reasons for not prioritising social engagement. Think about your typical weekly schedule, noting when you usually have free time and feel you could socialise. This way, you can plan ahead and make space for social activities.

8. Reach out: Don't wait for others to make plans. Reach out to friends or family for a catch-up or a coffee. Reconnecting with people can boost your sense of social connection.

9. Go to events: Even if you're not feeling up to it, push yourself to attend events you're invited to. It can help increase social connection, and if you don't find it that much fun, you can reward yourself afterwards for being brave enough to go out.

10. Step out of your comfort zone: Be open to meeting new people and trying new things. Start conversations with those around you and be patient as you build new connections.

11. Practice active listening: When you're talking with others, focus on truly listening and showing interest. Ask questions and be friendly to make interactions more engaging. Maintain a positive and approachable demeanour, smile, and make eye contact. Displaying warmth and friendliness can make it easier for others to engage with you socially.

Step Six Checklist: Social Engagement

Social engagement is a big deal when it comes to your mental health, and it's awesome that you're equipped to make some changes. Here's a checklist to help you make the most of your social interactions and boost your mental wellbeing:

☐ **Understand the basics:** Make sure you've read through the social engagement tips and really get the ideas behind them.

☐ **Everyday chats:** Try to strike up conversations in your daily life more often than usual.

☐ **In-person meet-ups:** When you can, choose face-to-face interactions over virtual ones.

☐ **Host friends or family:** Invite people over to your place for a get-together.

☐ **Join activities:** Find a group or activity you haven't tried before and get involved.

☐ **Plan social time:** Set aside specific times in your calendar for social activities.

☐ **Reach out:** Don't wait for others to contact you—take the initiative to get in touch first.

☐ **Attend events:** Go to social gatherings you're invited to, even if you're not sure you want to.

☐ **Listen actively:** Really focus on listening when you're talking with others.

☐ **Move forward:** Once you've got an understanding of this step, you can tackle the self-care and hobbies step.

Step Seven:
Self-Care and Hobbies

You can't run on empty! In other words, it is important to find time to do something that reminds you that you matter. We need to look after ourselves, and self-care and hobbies form a large part of that care.

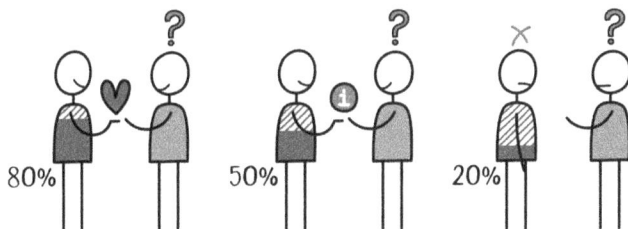

Self-care and hobbies leave us feeling relaxed, energised, and refreshed. When was the last time you engaged in something that left you feeling this way?

In this step, we'll explore how self-care and hobbies are linked to mental health and go over some easy, practical ways you can boost your self-care and get more involved in the hobbies you enjoy.

Dr Kaylee Crockett, a clinical psychologist at the University of Alabama at Birmingham, says that doing things we enjoy and taking care of ourselves is crucial for our wellbeing. These activities help us stay connected to who we are and what's important to us. They're not just good for mental health, but they can also help us live healthier lives, bounce back from tough times, and even reduce healthcare costs.

For many of us, finding time for exercise or social activities can be tough, so we might overlook the importance of self-care and hobbies. Instead of seeing these activities as luxuries or rewards, it's helpful to think of them as essential parts of our daily routine, especially when we're facing mental health challenges. Taking care of ourselves and engaging in activities we love helps build a strong relationship with ourselves, which is key to overall wellbeing. Self-care and hobbies are vital for nurturing that relationship.

How will self-care and hobbies boost my mental health?

Even small acts of self-care or spending time on hobbies each day can make a big difference. Doing activities you enjoy and taking care of yourself can help you feel better both physically and mentally. It's important to make time for these activities as part of your overall wellbeing because they can have a positive impact on your mental health in many different ways.

Reduced stress: Self-care and hobbies help us manage stress because they are fun and promote rest and relaxation, according to a study by Dr Elkin Luis from the University of Navarra.

Improved mood: Self-care and hobbies release feel-good endorphins and dopamine into our brains, which lifts our mood according to practising psychiatrist and author Dr Gregory Brown.

Coping mechanism: Taking care of ourselves and diving into hobbies can be a great way to handle stress and keep our emotions in check. A study by Dr Elkin Luis from the University of Navarra, which looked at over 1,000 people, found that these activities can really help improve our mental health.

Balance: Doing things we enjoy outside of life commitments helps bring more balance to our lives. It's like hitting the reset button and improving our overall wellbeing.

Self-identity: Trying out new interests or reconnecting with old ones helps us understand ourselves better beyond just our daily responsibilities. It's a great way to build a stronger sense of who we are.

Prevention: Regular self-care and hobbies aren't just for relaxation—they also help reduce stress and improve our mood. This ongoing practice can be a good way to prevent mental health issues such as depression and anxiety from developing.

Presence: Think about times you have been engaging in a self-care activity or hobby. I know from my own experience that I am more likely to be focused on that self-care activity than on outside responsibilities. When we're engaged in a self-care activity or hobby, we're more likely to be focused on that than be stressing over daily responsibilities. This focus acts as mindfulness, helping us stay present and enjoy the moment. For instance, a relaxing massage might help us forget our work stress, unlike sitting on the couch and ruminating.

Emotional expression: Many hobbies and self-care activities, such as painting or journalling, help us express our emotions. This can make it easier to handle challenges and build resilience against stress.

Self-compassion: Engaging in activities that care for and nurture us naturally fosters self-compassion. It's a way of treating ourselves with kindness and understanding.

Case study:

After my client, Alex, noticed high stress levels and burnout, we reviewed his typical weekly schedule. On paper, it became obvious that he wasn't making any time for self-care or hobbies. I suggested he start setting aside time each week for activities he enjoyed, such as playing guitar and gardening. Within a few weeks of incorporating these hobbies into his routine, Alex felt much more relaxed and balanced. This simple shift in focus helped him manage stress better and improved his overall wellbeing.

What self-care forms are there?

Self-care is all about intentionally taking time for practices that boost our physical, mental, and emotional health. It means making ourselves a priority and choosing activities that help us relax, reduce stress, and feel good overall.

Finding what works for you is key—whether it's a soothing bath, a good book, or a walk in nature. The idea is to pick activities that make you feel better and fit your needs.

A study by Dr Lisa Butler suggests self-care should touch on 6 areas of life: physical, professional, relational, emotional, psychological, and spiritual. Paying attention to each of these areas can bring extra benefits and a more balanced approach to self-care.

Remember, self-care is personal and what works best for one person might be different for another. So, find what suits you and makes you feel great!

What hobbies can I do?

Hobbies are activities we do just for fun, relaxation, and personal satisfaction. They let us get creative, learn new skills, and take a break from our daily grind. Trying out different hobbies can help us find what we truly enjoy and boost our overall happiness. There are 4 main types of hobbies to consider: physical, intellectual, creative, and community focused.

Physical hobbies

Physical hobbies are activities that get you moving and help boost your fitness and overall health. They're not just good for your body but also great for fun and relaxation.

Common examples:

- gardening
- hiking or nature walks
- dancing
- swimming, running, and cycling
- camping
- Pilates and yoga
- birdwatching
- rock climbing
- team sports
- kayaking or canoeing
- martial arts
- meditation, mindfulness practices, and breathing exercises
- tai chi

Intellectual hobbies

Intellectual hobbies are activities that challenge your brain and help you learn new things. They're all about thinking, problem-solving, and expanding your knowledge in areas that interest you.

Common examples:

- reading (including this guide)
- learning a new language
- studying or researching
- completing online courses or workshops
- collecting (e.g. coins, stamps, antiques, memorabilia, art, books)
- puzzle-solving (e.g. crossword puzzles, jigsaw puzzles)
- trivia or quiz nights
- board games or card games
- escape-room challenges
- learning about science or technology advancements

- blogging and podcasting
- building and repairing electronics
- astronomy

Creative hobbies

Creative hobbies are all about using your imagination and expressing yourself artistically. They let you explore new ideas and innovate in fun and personal ways.

Common examples:

- cooking and baking with new recipes
- experimenting with different cuisines
- photography
- painting and drawing
- writing
- playing a musical instrument, DJing, singing, or composing music
- do-it-yourself projects
- crafting
- sculpting
- graphic design
- furniture restoration
- interior design

Community hobbies

Community hobbies are activities that get you interacting with others and working together. They're great for building relationships, feeling connected, and giving back to your community.

Common examples:

- organising events or parties
- hosting game nights or movie nights
- joining discussion groups

- volunteering
- book clubs
- joining local sporting teams
- following sports teams
- travelling and exploring new places
- joining local land-care groups

How do I optimise my self-care and hobby practices?

Incorporating self-care and hobbies into our daily routines is crucial for our overall wellbeing—physical, mental, and emotional. Keep in mind that what works for you might be different from what works for others. The important thing is to regularly prioritise these activities and make them a consistent part of our lives. Experts from the University of Alabama at Birmingham's Department of Family and Community Medicine suggest that we make time for self-care and hobbies and protect that time intentionally. Here are some strategies to help you do just that:

1. Keep up with self-care and hobbies: Self-care and hobbies can be fun. They also need effort and if we're not feeling our best, can be forgotten or seem like too much trouble. If you've followed the earlier steps in this guide, you might be feeling ready enough to dive back into these activities and enjoy them.

2. Identify what's holding you back: Research shows that recognising what's holding you back is crucial for making changes. Take a moment to reflect on why you're not engaging in more self-care or hobbies. Once you pinpoint these barriers, think about how you can lessen their impact. For example, for me it was as simple as not allocating a consistent time slot each week for myself.

3. Start small with achievable goals: Change is easier when you start small. Begin with simple self-care and hobby activities you can easily fit into your routine, and gradually build up to more involved practices. Aimee Daramus, a licensed clinical psychologist, suggests finding quick activities that can be done in 5 minutes or less if needed.

4. Make a self-care and hobby menu: Make a list of self-care activities and hobbies you enjoy or might like to try. This list can be a handy reference when you're looking for something to do. I have one of these in the notes on my phone, including a mixture of regular favourites and new activities to try.

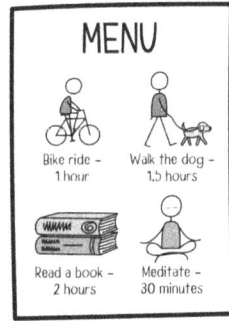

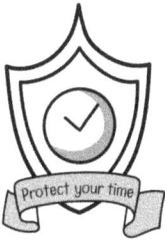

5. Limit distractions: Dr Kaylee Crockett, a clinical psychologist, recommends taking steps to minimise distractions while engaging in self-care and hobbies. Turn your phone on "do not disturb" and let others know you're unavailable during this time. This helps you fully enjoy the activity.

6. Explore new activities: We often stick to what we know, but trying new things can be rewarding. Psychologists suggest activity sampling, which means regularly experimenting with new self-care practices or hobbies to discover new interests.

7. Plan your self-care and hobbies time: According to Dr Alyson Ross from the National Institutes of Health Clinical Center, a common barrier to engaging in self-care and hobbies is not having enough time. We always seem to have time for work even though it consumes the most active hours of our week yet run out of time for self-care and hobbies. Ask yourself, "Why is this the case?" We just do not prioritise ourselves enough. Reflect on your average week's schedule and think of times you usually have free time slots. Set aside some of these for self-care and hobbies and plan specific activities for these times.

8. Set clear boundaries for personal time: Part of the reason people find time for work, but not for their self-care and hobbies, is due to contractual agreements they have with their workplace, which set clear boundaries and expectations. If you set these same boundaries for yourself and learn to say no to unnecessary requests and commitments, you will protect your time and energy and make self-care and hobbies time non-negotiable.

9. Start your day with self-care or a hobby: Start your day with a self-care activity or hobby to set a positive tone. This could be morning meditation, stretching, or a walk. For me, it's sipping lemon water in the sun, which keeps me off my phone and helps regulate my body's sleep rhythm while hydrating me.

Step Seven Checklist: Self-Care and Hobbies

You should now see how essential self-care and hobbies are for your mental health and feel confident in applying strategies to increase your engagement in these activities. This checklist is designed to help you successfully incorporate self-care and hobbies into your life to improve your mental wellbeing. Following these steps will ensure you get the most out of this process:

☐ **Review self-care and hobbies:** Make sure you understand the concepts and benefits of self-care and hobbies by reviewing the information thoroughly.

☐ **Identify and address barriers:** Think about what might be preventing you from engaging in self-care and hobbies and find ways to reduce these barriers.

☐ **Start small and simple:** Begin with a hobby or self-care activity that takes just 5 to 10 minutes.

☐ **Self-care and hobby list:** Write down and print out a list of activities you enjoy or want to try.

☐ **Reduce distractions:** Take steps to minimise any distractions during your self-care or hobby time.

☐ **Explore new activities:** Try out different hobbies or self-care practices to see what you like.

☐ **Schedule regular time:** Set a specific time each week dedicated to self-care or hobbies.

☐ **Set clear boundaries:** Make sure to protect your self-care and hobbies time by setting boundaries and saying no when necessary.

☐ **Establish a morning routine:** Start each day with a quick, 5-minute self-care activity or hobby.

☐ **Advance to the next step:** Once you have these practices in place, move on to the digital detox step.

Step Eight: Digital Detox

In this step, focused on digital detox, we'll explore how screen time affects our mental health and share some easy, practical tips to help you cut down on your screen use and feel better overall.

Recent data from 2024 shows that *the average person now spends nearly 7 hours a day on screens connected to the internet,* which is a full hour more than just 10 years ago. For Gen Z, that number jumps to about 9 hours a day!

To give you a clearer picture, research by Sudheer Kumar Muppalla from the Institute of Medical Sciences suggests that *adults should ideally spend no more than 2 hours a day on screens for non-work-related activities* to maintain good health. But in reality, most people are spending about 250% more time on screens than recommended.

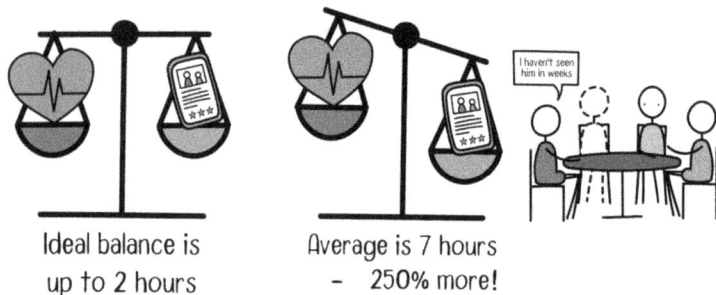

Ideal balance is
up to 2 hours

Average is 7 hours
– 250% more!

Think of it like this: if the average person consumed 250% more calories than they should each day, we'd see a huge increase in health problems. While spending too much time on screens might not show obvious physical signs like overeating might, it can still have serious effects on our mental and emotional wellbeing. Because these effects aren't as immediately noticeable as physical symptoms, we tend not to take them as seriously, which can make the problem worse.

By being mindful of our screen time and making small changes, we can start to see improvements in our mental health and overall happiness.

How will reducing screen time boost my mental health?

The effect of screen use on mental health can vary depending on factors like content type and individual sensitivity. However, reducing your screen time, even a little each day, can significantly improve your mental wellbeing. Prioritising less screen time is an important part of maintaining overall health and can benefit your mental health in the following ways:

Better sleep: Screens emit blue light, which interferes with sleep patterns, and so reducing our use of them promotes our circadian sleep rhythm, according to a study by Daneyal Arshad from Rawalpindi Medical University.

More face-to-face interactions: Spending too much time on digital devices often means we miss out on real-life interactions.

According to the Digital Health Task Force in Ottawa, Canada, reducing screen time can boost the amount of face-to-face time we get with others.

Extra free time: On average, we spend about 7 hours a day on digital devices, and about the same amount sleeping. That leaves us with just 10 hours for everything else, which isn't much if you're working. Cutting back on screen time could free up more hours for hobbies, exercise, and relaxation.

Increased physical activity: Too much screen time can lead to less physical activity. However, according to Dr Allana LeBlanc from the University of Ottawa Heart Institute healthier amounts of screen time are linked to more active lifestyles.

Lower stress: Excessive screen time, especially on social media, is strongly linked to higher stress levels. A review of 15 studies by Apriana Rahmawati found that spending more than 2 hours a day on screens can increase stress by reducing time for relaxing activities, disrupting sleep, and exposing you to negative information. Cutting back on your screen time can help ease these stressors and give your mind a break.

Breaking screen addiction: An average daily screen time of more than 2 hours is positively associated with screen and social media addiction, according to the research of Apriana Rahmawati. Since many of us average around 7 hours a day, it's no surprise that screen addiction is common. Reducing screen time can help break this cycle and promote healthier habits.

Improved mental health: The less time you spend on digital devices, the lower your risk of mental health issues, according to a review by Abida Sultana from the Nature Study Society of Bangladesh.

Finding balance: Minimising screen time means more time for real-life connections, exercise, and other fulfilling activities. By cutting down on screen time, you can find a better balance and prioritise activities that benefit your mental and physical health.

Enhanced presence and productivity: Spending 7 hours a day on screens can lead to constant distractions and reduced productivity. By limiting your screen time, you can become more present, engage more fully in life, and boost your overall productivity.

Case study:

I decided to cut back on my screen time after tracking revealed I was spending much more than the suggested 2 hours on screens per day. I started by leaving my phone in the car when I went out for dinner or at home when exercising. This small change helped me stay more present and enjoy these activities fully. Within a few weeks, I noticed I felt more connected at dinner and more relaxed after the workouts. It made a notable difference in my overall sense of wellbeing.

How do I reduce my screen time?

Every minute you cut back on screen time can benefit your mental health, so even small changes are progress! Reducing your screen time doesn't mean you have to eliminate digital devices from your life. The key is to be more mindful about how much time you're spending on screens. The goal is to aim to get closer to the recommended limit of 2 hours per day, instead of the current average of 7 hours. Here are some strategies to help reduce your screen time:

1. Follow the earlier steps of this guide: Reducing your screen time gives you more free time, and the earlier steps in this guide have suggested activities like self-care, hobbies, and exercise that take up time. If you're doing these activities, you'll naturally have less time to spend on digital devices. Well done!

2. Track your screen time: Most phones, tablets, and laptops have features to track screen time. On an iPhone, you can check this in your settings in under a minute. If you're not sure how to find this on your device, look up a guide online. Don't forget to include time spent watching TV or using other screens. Add it up and compare it to the average of 7 hours a day and the recommended 2 hours. Keeping track helps you see how much you need to cut back. I was shocked at my own accumulation here!

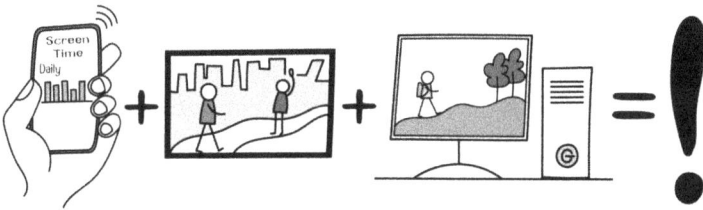

3. Start small with realistic goals: When making any change, it's best to start small. For example, try not to use your phone until 9 am each day. This way, you're not overwhelmed by a big change right away.

4. Turn off notifications: Apps constantly ask if you want notifications because it keeps you coming back. Research including that of Abhinav Mehrotra, shows that notifications increase our phone use and can trigger dopamine release, which can lead to addiction. Turning them off helps reduce usage and lowers the risk of becoming addicted to your devices.

5. Set time limits: You can now set time limits for specific apps. Once you hit the limit, the app locks, helping you monitor your screen time in real time and cut down on overuse. I use this feature myself on a couple of apps, which my tracking of screen time suggested I was overusing.

6. Remove unnecessary apps: Delete 1 or 2 apps that you tend to overuse and see how you feel. You might find that you unlock your phone out of habit, only to put it down again when you realise the app is gone. This shows how much you relied on those apps. Again, I found myself doing this and it was a concerning realisation.

7. Create screen-free zones: Designate certain areas in your home as screen-free, for example, by keeping your bedroom free of TV and charging your phone in another room. This reduces the temptation to check your phone constantly.

8. Take breaks: Make sure to schedule times throughout your day when you're not using any digital devices. Even short breaks can help reduce the overall impact of screen time.

9. Find other activities: Boredom often leads to more screen time and even addiction, according to research led by Yali Zhang of Renmin University in China. By filling your day with meaningful activities, such as hobbies or socialising, you'll feel more engaged and less likely to turn to your phone.

10. Set boundaries: Force yourself to be without your devices in certain situations. For instance, leave your phone in the car when you go out for dinner or at home when you go for a walk. If you need to pay for things, use cash or a card instead of your phone.

11. Use blue-light filters: Too much blue light can mess with your sleep and mental health. A study by Dr Kimberly Burkhart of the University of Toledo found that people who used blue-light-blocking glasses experienced major improvements in both sleep quality and mood. You can also use other blue-light filters, but glasses are often the easiest option.

12. Start a morning ritual: Begin your day by getting out of bed without looking at your phone and spend 15 minutes outside in the sunlight. This can help counteract the negative effects of screen exposure and regulate your sleep cycle.

13. Engage in offline activities: Plan activities that don't involve screens, such as playing board games, reading, cooking, or spending time outdoors.

14. Tell others about your plan: Let your friends, family, and co-workers know you're trying to cut back on your screen time. This helps them understand why you might not respond right away and reduces any pressure you might feel.

15. Build a support system: Get friends or family involved in your effort to reduce screen time, or at least let them know when you're having screen-free moments, so they can support you.

16. Reflect and evaluate: After spending less time on your devices, think about how it feels and how it has affected your mental and emotional wellbeing. Reflect on your experience, especially after specific detox periods, such as leaving your phone at home during a dinner out.

Step Eight Checklist: Digital Detox

By now, you should understand the benefits of reducing your digital device use and feel ready to start reducing your screen time. Use this checklist to help you detox from digital devices or cut back on your usage. Following these steps will help you make the most of this process:

☐ **Read the digital detox content:** Make sure you've gone over the digital detox section and understand the key points.

☐ **Track your screen time:** Keep an eye on how much time you're spending on your devices.

☐ **Turn off notifications:** Disable notifications for all apps to reduce distractions.

☐ **Set app time limits:** Set limits on the time you spend on apps that you use too much.

☐ **Delete unnecessary apps:** Remove apps from your phone that you don't need or overuse.

☐ **Create screen-free zones:** Set up areas in your home where screens aren't allowed, such as your bedroom.

☐ **Take breaks:** Make sure to take regular breaks when using digital devices.

☐ **Find other activities:** Schedule activities to do during times when you might feel bored.

☐ **Set boundaries:** Create rules for yourself, such as leaving your phone in the car when you're out for dinner.

☐ **Use blue-light filters:** Get blue-light-blocking glasses or filters to protect your eyes.

☐ **Morning routine:** Start your mornings without using any digital devices.

☐ **Do offline activities:** Plan activities that don't involve screens, such as reading a book or playing board games.

☐ **Tell others:** Let people know you're cutting back on screen time, so they understand if you don't respond right away.

☐ **Reflect on your progress:** Take time to think about how these changes are affecting you.

☐ **Move to the next step:** When you're ready, move on to the gratitude step.

Step Nine:
Gratitude

In this step, we're going to explore how gratitude can improve our mental health and look at some simple, practical ways to make it a part of our daily lives.

Harvard researcher Shawn Achor reports that ***writing down just 3 things you're grateful for every day for 21 days can rewire your brain*** and boost your optimism significantly, and the benefits last for 6 months!

Research from the University of Pennsylvania, led by Martin Seligman and cited over 10,000 times, shows that actively practising gratitude can lower stress, anxiety, and depression. In fact, just ***one small act of gratitude can make you 10% happier and reduce symptoms of depression by 35%.***

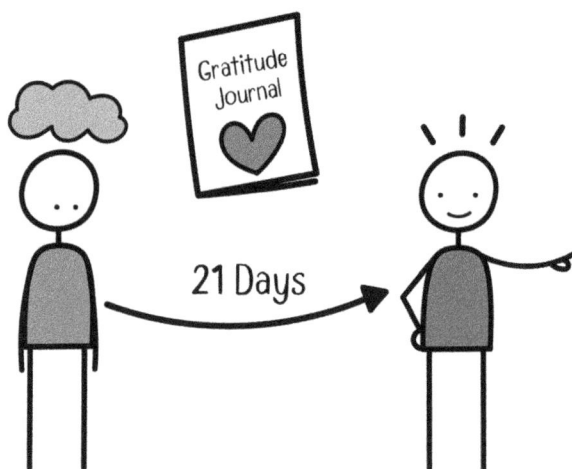

Think about it—just 2 minutes a day to write down something you're grateful for can dramatically reduce negative feelings and give you a quick boost in happiness. It's like a free, easy-to-use antidepressant!

Gratitude is simply our way of recognising the good things in life. Psychologists define it as a positive emotional response when we notice and appreciate what we have. The Mindfulness Awareness Research Center at the University of California, Los Angeles, has found solid evidence supporting the benefits of gratitude. *Advanced brain imaging has shown that engaging in gratitude can change the brain's structure*, making us feel happier and more content. Gratitude activates the brain's reward centre, which shifts how we see ourselves and the world around us. Dr Alex Korb also points out that practising gratitude helps us focus on the positive aspects of our lives.

How will gratitude boost my mental health?

Although gratitude is discussed some way through this guide, its impact is just as impressive as the earlier steps. Once you start following the earlier steps, you'll have even more to be thankful for, which makes practising gratitude easier. Gratitude affects a bunch of different parts of our mental health.

Boosted mood chemicals: Gratitude increases the release of neurotransmitters tied to happiness and mood. Dr Hongbo Yu from Peking University found that feeling grateful actually increases the release of dopamine and serotonin.

Activated brain areas: A team from Indiana University, led by Prathik Kini, did brain scans before and after people practised gratitude. They found that gratitude lights up areas of the brain connected to reward, empathy, and emotions. And the best part? These positive effects were seen for up to 3 months.

Improved sleep quality: Dr Anna Boggiss and her team at the University of Auckland reviewed 19 studies to see how gratitude affects health and found that being grateful can really help improve how well you sleep.

Lowered stress levels: Practising gratitude can lower stress hormones such as cortisol, which helps reduce stress. Professor Murat Yıldırım from the University of Leicester found that people who are more grateful tend to feel more satisfied with life because they experience less stress.

Better physical health: Dr Robert Emmons, a psychology professor at University of California Davis, found that gratitude not only boosts overall health but also leads to better health habits. Grateful people often eat better, exercise more, and have other healthy behaviours. Plus, they have stronger immune systems, lower blood pressure, and less inflammation.

Enhanced mindfulness: Gratitude is a way of being mindful— it helps you stay present and appreciate the good things in your life. By focusing on what's positive, gratitude can clear your mind and ease anxiety about the past or future. Gratitude also shifts your focus from what you feel your life is lacking or what is negative to what is abundant and positive.

Case study:

In 2017, Australian Football League (AFL) star Dustin Martin felt lost and experienced some unwanted mental health symptoms. For those outside of Australia, AFL football is our national sport, and Dustin Martin is one of the greatest ever players to play the game. Dustin began using The Resilience Project's journal, which focuses on gratitude, mindfulness, and empathy. This tool helped him stay calm and centred during a high-pressure season. Martin credited the journal with enhancing his mental clarity and appreciation, contributing to his record-setting AFL Brownlow Medal win (the highest individual award a player can win) with 36 votes. By integrating daily reflections into his routine, Martin improved his performance and overall wellbeing, showcasing gratitude's positive impact.

What gratitude forms are there?

There are lots of ways to practise gratitude, allowing you to choose the method or methods that best fit you and your life. Try some out and see what suits you best. This might involve trial and error.

Gratitude journalling: Write down things you are grateful for regularly, ideally daily, weekly, or as often as you like. This practice encourages reflection on positive aspects of your life.

Three good things: Each day, identify and jot down 3 things that went well or made you feel grateful. Reflect on why these events or experiences made you thankful. Incorporate this during your sit-down dinner with yourself or your friends or family.

Blessing count: Set aside a specific time each day to count your blessings. Literally count them, ideally via writing them down, and focus on the details of each one.

Gratitude letters or message: Write a letter or message to someone important to you, expressing your gratitude and appreciation for them. You can choose to send it or keep it as a personal reflection.

Gratitude jar: Place a jar in a central location in your home and leave slips of paper nearby. Whenever you feel grateful for something, write it down on a slip and put it in the jar. Review the notes periodically or do this as a household and read a couple each dinnertime.

Gratitude meditation: Incorporate gratitude into your meditation practice. During your meditation, focus on feelings of gratitude and appreciation. You can use guided gratitude meditation scripts or apps for this purpose.

Mindful gratitude: Engage in daily activities mindfully, paying attention to the details and being grateful for the sensory experiences. For example, savour the aroma of your morning coffee or appreciate the warmth of the sun on your skin.

Gratitude walks: During a walk or hike, consciously focus on the beauty of nature—the sights, sounds, and sensations. Express gratitude for the opportunity to connect with the natural world.

Gratitude affirmations: Gratitude affirmations are positive statements that reinforce your feelings of gratitude. Repeat them regularly to cultivate a grateful mindset.

Random acts of kindness: Perform acts of kindness for others without expecting anything in return. The act of giving can generate feelings of gratitude.

Visual gratitude board: Create a physical or digital gratitude board filled with images, quotes, and reminders of what you are grateful for. Review it regularly.

Gratitude apps: Use mobile apps specifically designed for gratitude practices. These apps often provide prompts, reminders, and a structured way to engage in gratitude exercises.

Avoid comparison: Avoid comparing your life to others', especially on social media. Instead, focus on your own journey and the unique blessings it brings.

Celebrate milestones: When you achieve a goal or reach a milestone, celebrate it with gratitude. Recognise the hard work and support that contributed to your success.

How do I increase my gratitude practices?

Adding gratitude to your daily routine can really boost your mental health. Keep in mind that gratitude looks different for everyone—it's all about finding what feels right for you. The goal is to focus on the positive parts of your life. Over time, this can help shift your mindset to be more positive and appreciative, bringing a bunch of great benefits. Here are some tips to help you weave gratitude into your life:

1. Build on what you've already started: If you've been following the earlier steps of this guide, you're already on the right track. As you continue, you'll find more things to be grateful for, and practising gratitude will start to feel more natural.

2. Start small and keep it simple: Research led by Professor Sonja Lyubomirsky from the University of California suggests that keeping gratitude simple is key. As with any new habit, it's best to start with small steps. Choose gratitude practices that are easy for you to fit into your daily life.

3. Try different ways to express your gratitude: According to Professor Philip Watkins, trying out various forms of gratitude can help you stick with it. Experiment with different methods until you find what works best for you and fits into your lifestyle.

4. Find moments to be thankful throughout your day: Look for small opportunities to practise gratitude.

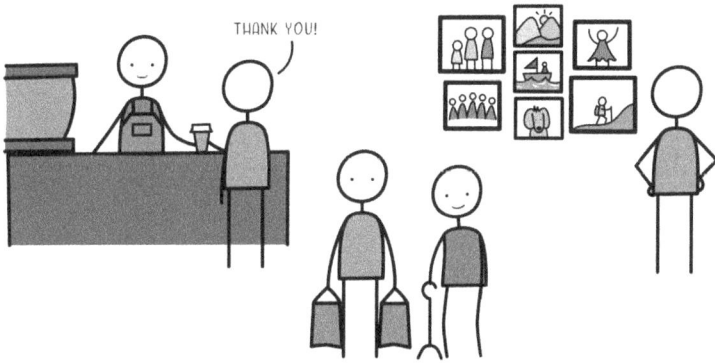

5. Make it part of your routine: Schedule a specific time for gratitude so you don't forget. You could make it a ritual, for example, sharing 2 things you're grateful for at the dinner table or enjoying your morning coffee while looking at your favourite photos. These routines can help turn gratitude into a habit.

6. Set reminders: Use your phone, calendar, or even sticky notes to remind yourself to practise gratitude. Alarms and alerts can give you a gentle nudge to stay on track and keep gratitude in your daily routine.

Step Nine Checklist: Gratitude

By now, you should see how important gratitude can be for your mental health, and hopefully, you feel ready to try some new ways to bring more gratitude into your life. This checklist is here to guide you in making gratitude a regular part of your routine, helping to boost your mental wellbeing. Follow these steps to make the most out of this practice:

☐ **Review the gratitude basics:** Make sure you've read through the gratitude section and feel comfortable with the ideas.

☐ **Start small:** Choose a gratitude practice that easily fits into your current lifestyle.

☐ **Experiment:** Try out different types of gratitude activities to find what feels right for you.

☐ **Incorporate gratitude into your day:** Look for ways to practise gratitude in your everyday life, like buying coffee for a stranger or thanking someone who helps you.

☐ **Create a schedule:** Set aside specific times in your day to focus on gratitude.

☐ **Set reminders:** Use reminders to help you stay consistent with your gratitude practice.

☐ **Move forward:** Once you've got this down, you're ready to move on to the cognitive behaviour therapy step.

Step Ten: Cognitive Behaviour Therapy

In this step we look at how to use cognitive behaviour therapy (CBT) techniques in simple, practical ways to promote your mental health.

Before we begin, it's important to know that CBT is most effective when administered by registered psychologists who have undergone years of education and supervised training. However, I understand that not everyone can access professional psychology services. That's why it's useful to have a basic understanding of some common CBT techniques that you can try at home.

CBT is one of the most used and well-researched types of therapy that psychologists use. It's known for being effective in treating various mental health issues. For example, a review of 269 published studies led by Dr Stefan Hofmann at Boston University found that CBT works exceptionally well for many mental health concerns and conditions, with strong positive results.

Another study, from Vanderbilt University led by Professor Steven Hollon, showed that **CBT is just as effective as antidepressants** for general mental health issues. Plus, people who recover from mental health challenges with CBT are less likely to relapse with symptoms compared with those who use medications. Brain scans from this research also shows that CBT helps your brain manage and regulate its activity, while medications usually focus on reducing the stress response and can sometimes be seen as a Band-Aid approach. A CBT approach is often preferred because it works by helping you address the root causes, which is also what this guide aims to help you achieve.

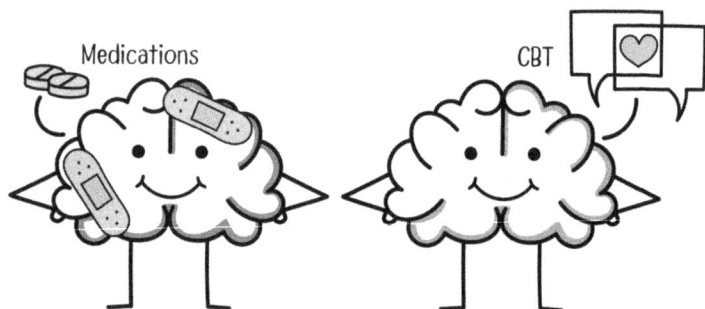

Medications   CBT

How will cognitive behaviour therapy boost my mental health?

Our thoughts shape our feelings, which then influence our actions and impact our lives. According to Dr Judith Beck of the University of Pennsylvania, these thoughts, feelings, and actions form a cycle in which each part affects the other parts. CBT helps us understand and break this cycle. According to Dr Jesse Wright of the University of Louisville, it does this using 2 main strategies:

- **Cognitive:** This strategy helps you identify and challenge negative thoughts and beliefs, and manage the emotions linked to them.
- **Behavioural:** This strategy focuses on changing the actions that come from negative thoughts and feelings.

The cycle of thoughts, feelings, and behaviours is often shown as a triangle, illustrating how they all connect.

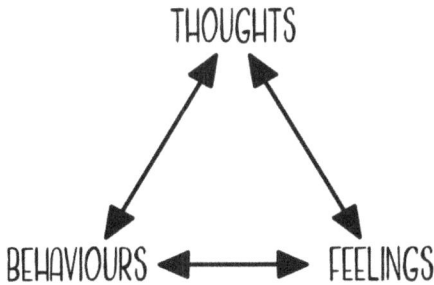

THOUGHTS

BEHAVIOURS ◄──► FEELINGS

Thoughts are our beliefs, attitudes, and expectations about ourselves, others, and the world. A 2020 study by Julie Tseng at Queen's University found that people have over 6,000 thoughts daily, both good and bad. When these thoughts become unbalanced, we might feel negative emotions and act in ways that are risky or that avoid helpful behaviours. CBT helps by changing our thoughts to restore balance, which can improve our feelings and actions. For instance, replacing "I always mess up" with "I can improve with practice" can boost confidence and encourage us to try new things.

Feelings are emotional responses to our thoughts and situations; these include happiness, sadness, and anxiety. These emotions can impact how we think and act. For instance, feeling anxious might lead you to think "This is too hard" and avoid challenging tasks such as learning a new skill. CBT helps by improving our ability to manage emotions, leading to healthier behaviours and more positive thoughts. For example, CBT can help us replace "This is too hard" with "I can handle this", making us more likely to face challenges confidently.

Behaviours are our actions or reactions to things happening around us or inside our minds, sometimes manifesting as habits and routines. They can reinforce our thoughts and feelings. For example, avoiding a challenging situation can make us believe it's too hard and keep us feeling anxious. CBT helps by encouraging us to engage in positive, healthy behaviours, which can boost our mood and lead to more positive thoughts.

Case study:

John had struggled with anxiety and low self-esteem for years. After starting CBT with me, he committed to the process for 8 weeks. Through targeted exercises and changing negative thought patterns, John experienced a dramatic shift. He improved his self-confidence, managed stress better, and began setting and achieving personal goals. By the end of the therapy and under the guidance of his GP, John began reducing his antidepressant dose, so profound was the effect of CBT.

Thought-based forms of cognitive behaviour therapy

CBT is tailored to your unique experiences and needs, helping you manage negative thoughts (such as thinking in extremes, expecting the worst, or making broad generalisations) by first identifying them through thought records—where you track your negative thoughts, their triggers, and their emotional and physical impact. Next, you challenge these thoughts using cognitive restructuring to determine if they are based on facts or assumptions. Finally, you replace them with more balanced and positive perspectives through reframing. This process helps shift your thinking to a more realistic and constructive outlook when you catch yourself having negative thoughts. You can try this process yourself by following these steps:

1. Situation: Write down what happened that triggered your negative reaction. For example, you see a friend's social media post about a fun event you weren't invited to.

2. Negative thought: Write down the negative thought you had because of the situation. For example, "They must not like me anymore; I'm not important to them."

3. Emotional response: Write down the feelings caused by the negative thought. For example, sad, rejected, or left out.

4. Physical sensation: Write down the sensations in your body caused by your emotional response. For example, you might feel a heaviness in your chest or a lump in your throat.

5. Question the thought/evidence: Write down questions to help you examine the thought and any evidence that supports or contradicts it. For example, "Is this thought based on actual facts, or am I assuming they don't like me just because I wasn't invited?" (question), "I wasn't invited to this event" (supporting evidence), "They invited me to their birthday last month, and we've been texting this week" (contradicting evidence).

6. Change the thought: Write down a more balanced thought after examining the evidence and use positive self-talk to reinforce this new thought. For example, "Just because I wasn't invited to this one event doesn't mean they don't like me. There could be many reasons I wasn't included, and it doesn't define our friendship. I have good friends who care about me, and missing one event doesn't change that. I can reach out and make plans with them another time."

CBT Worksheet

Situation	
Negative thought	
Emotional response	
Physical sensation	
Question the thought/evidence	
Change the thought	

Feelings-based forms of cognitive behaviour therapy

Now that you know what triggers your negative thoughts and feelings, it's time to focus on managing your emotions using mindfulness and emotion regulation. Mindfulness helps you observe and accept your thoughts and feelings without getting overwhelmed, making it easier to understand them. Emotion regulation techniques then help you manage and respond to these feelings more effectively. Experiment with these simple techniques to help you navigate your emotions, especially the negative ones:

Deep breathing: Breathe slowly and deeply to relax. Inhale for 4 seconds, hold for 4 seconds, and exhale for 4 seconds. Repeat this cycle for 2 minutes.

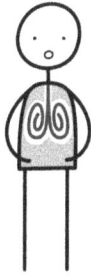

Inhale for 4 seconds
Hold for 4 seconds
Exhale for 4 seconds
Repeat for 2 minutes

Progressive muscle relaxation: Tense and then relax different muscle groups. Tense your fists for 5 seconds, then relax them for 10 seconds. Move to your shoulders, tense for 5 seconds, then relax for 10 seconds. Repeat with each muscle group.

Mindfulness meditation: Pay attention to your thoughts and feelings without judgement. Sit comfortably and focus on your breath. Notice each inhalation and exhalation without judgement. If your mind wanders, gently bring your attention back to your breath. Do this for 2 minutes.

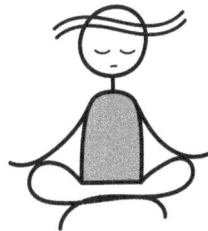

Guided imagery: Visualise a calm, peaceful place. Close your eyes and imagine a peaceful place, such as a beach or a forest. Picture the details—hear the sound of waves and smell the pine trees. Spend 2 minutes immersing yourself in this calming scene.

Sensory grounding: Redirect your focus to the present via the senses. Identify 5 things you can see, 4 things you can touch, 3 things you can hear, 2 things you can smell, and 1 thing you can taste.

Behaviour-based forms of cognitive behaviour therapy

Behaviour-based CBT helps you identify and change unhelpful actions. By adjusting these behaviours, CBT aims to break the cycle of negative thoughts and feelings, leading to healthier habits and better mental health. Try different behaviour-based CBT practices to see which ones work best for you—it might take some experimentation.

Behavioural activation: Plan and engage in activities you find meaningful to counteract low mood and inactivity. For example, if you enjoy reading, schedule time each week to read your favourite book. If you like spending time outdoors, plan a walk in the park or a gardening session.

Habit stacking: Habit stacking pairs a new habit with an existing one for a smoother routine. To implement it, pick a current habit and add a new, simple one right after. For example, if you drink lemon water every morning, stack on a new habit such as drinking it outside in the sun while barefoot. This not only helps you remember the new habit but also enhances mental health, regulates your sleep cycle, and provides grounding benefits.

Activity scheduling: Plan and structure daily activities to ensure a balanced and engaging routine, helping to combat depression and enhance overall wellbeing.

Contingency management: Use rewards or consequences to reinforce positive behaviours and discourage unhelpful ones. For example, reward yourself with a small treat after completing a challenging task. I use this all the time, sometimes to the extreme—following my successful completion of a degree I took myself to Asia for 3 weeks.

Activity monitoring: Track your daily activities, including your mood before and after each activity. This helps identify which activities have a positive or negative impact on your mental health.

Graded task assignment: Gradually expose yourself to activities that you perceive as challenging to help build confidence and reduce avoidance behaviours associated with low mood. Break down problems into manageable steps and evaluate potential solutions.

Exposure therapy: Gradually face and confront fears or anxiety-provoking situations to reduce avoidance and increase comfort. For instance, if you're afraid of flying, start by looking at pictures of aeroplanes and gradually work up to booking a short flight.

How do I engage in my own, personalised cognitive behaviour therapy?

Using CBT can be a helpful addition to your mental health routine and prepare you for working with a psychologist if you choose to. Even if you decide not to see a psychologist, these basic CBT techniques can still be useful. Keep in mind that CBT can be personalised, so focus on the particular methods that help you break your cycle of negative thoughts, feelings, and behaviours. Here are some strategies to try:

1. Follow the earlier steps: Use the techniques from the earlier parts of this guide to help manage your thoughts, feelings, and behaviours. While CBT often works best with a trained psychologist, starting with these steps will help you get ready for more advanced strategies.

2. Understand this step: Take the time to really comprehend this part so you get a solid grasp of how CBT works and its benefits. Knowing the theory can make the practice more effective and help you stay committed.

3. Start small and set realistic goals: Avy Joseph's CBT book (see Research Overview section) emphasises the power of small steps. Begin with 1 or 2 techniques and get comfortable with them before adding more. This way, you won't feel overwhelmed.

4. Make a schedule: Plan specific times for your CBT practices so you don't forget. Maybe set aside an hour or two each week to decide which techniques you'll use and how you'll do them. Writing this down on a whiteboard or in a diary can help make it a habit.

5. Use tools and resources: Take advantage of this book, along with apps and worksheets, to track your CBT progress. These tools can offer structure and keep you on track. My 2 personal favourite books, which I highly recommend, are: *Declutter Your Mind: How to Stop Worrying, Relieve Anxiety, and Eliminate Negative Thinking* (S.J. Scott and Barrie Davenport) and *Cognitive Behavioural Therapy: 7 Ways to Freedom from Anxiety, Depression, and Intrusive Thoughts* (Lawrence Wallace). My favourite CBT smart phone apps are called *Clarity: CBT Self Help Journal* and, for Apple users, *Bloom: CBT Therapy and Journal.*

6. Try different CBT methods: Experiment with various CBT techniques to find what works best for you. Mixing things up can make it easier to stick with the practice long-term.

7. Get feedback: Share your progress with a friend or a health professional to get their input and encouragement. Also, take some time to reflect on what's working for you.

8. Integrate CBT into your daily life: Look for chances to use CBT throughout your day. Try a quick mindfulness exercise while you're in the shower or plan an activity with a friend.

9. Set reminders: Use alarms, calendar alerts, or sticky notes to remind yourself to practise CBT. These little nudges can help you stay consistent in your practice.

10. Consider a psychologist: If you're not seeing improvements after following these steps, it might be time to consider getting support from a psychologist who can offer more structured guidance.

Step Ten Checklist: Cognitive Behaviour Therapy

Alright, so you're ready to dive into CBT and see how it can boost your mental health. Here's a handy checklist to help you get started and make the most of CBT:

- ☐ **Understand CBT:** Make sure you've got a good grasp of what CBT is all about. Give the main idea a read-through and check that you're clear on the basics.

- ☐ **Set goals:** Pick a small, manageable goal to start your CBT journey. It could be something simple like practising mindfulness for a few minutes each day.

- ☐ **Create a schedule:** Block out some time each week specifically for CBT activities. Consistency is key!

- ☐ **Use external tools:** Look for CBT apps or other tools that can help guide you through the process. There are some great resources out there.

- ☐ **Try different approaches:** Experiment with different CBT techniques to see what works best for you. It's okay to mix things up until you find your sweet spot.

- ☐ **Get feedback:** Chat with a trusted friend or family member about how you're using CBT. They might offer useful insights or encouragement.

- ☐ **Incorporate it daily:** Try to weave CBT into your everyday routine. For example, you might use your shower time to practise mindfulness.

- ☐ **Set reminders:** Make sure you have reminders set up so you don't forget your CBT sessions. Whether it's a phone alarm or a sticky note, find what works for you.

- ☐ **Consult a psychologist:** If you're still struggling despite your efforts, it might be helpful to see a registered psychologist for more support.

- ☐ **Explore extras:** Once you're comfortable with CBT, consider adding complementary approaches that could enhance your progress.

Complementary Approaches

In recent years, mental health treatment has expanded beyond traditional psychotherapy and medications to include alternative lifestyle treatments that go beyond just diet and exercise. These complementary approaches are gaining attention for their potential to boost overall wellbeing and even outperform conventional treatments in some cases.

For example, ice baths have shown promise in reducing unwanted mental health symptoms, while nature therapy, which involves spending time outdoors, has been found to improve mood, reduce stress, and enhance cognitive function.

In this step, we'll explore these and other complementary approaches. Keep in mind that these methods are varied and can offer different benefits. Some might work for you, and others might not, and that's perfectly okay. The goal is to experiment and find what best supports your mental health in a practical way.

This section will provide an overview of the most research-backed approaches, with practical tips on how to integrate them into your holistic mental health care plan. You will notice I haven't listed these approaches in any particular order, so feel free to try them out and see which ones resonate with you!

Celery juice

I know what you might be thinking: "Wasn't celery juice already mentioned in the nutrition step?" You're right, but its benefits are so impressive that it deserves another mention here!

I've been juicing celery myself for a couple of years now, and I notice without doubt the difference on the mornings I have it.

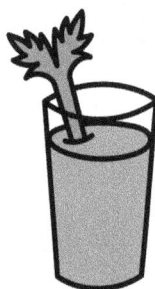

Celery juice is made by juicing fresh (preferably organic) celery or blending and straining the stalks to get the liquid. It's gained a lot of attention for its potential health perks, like boosting hydration, detoxifying the body, and reducing inflammation.

Celery is packed with vitamins A, C, and K, minerals including potassium and folate, and antioxidants that protect your cells from damage. It also contains unique compounds such as 3-n-butylphthalide, which can calm the nervous system, and luteolin, which helps produce neurotransmitters that are important for mental health.

A review of 9 studies led by Dr Wesam Kooti at the Kurdistan University of Medical Sciences looked at the impact of celery on mental health. It found that the antioxidants and anti-inflammatory compounds in celery reduce oxidative stress and inflammation, which are linked to mental health symptoms.

Case study:

After incorporating celery juice into my daily routine, I saw incredible improvements in both my physical and mental health. Within weeks, my digestion improved, and I felt more energetic. Mentally, I experienced enhanced focus and a boost in mood. This simple dietary change significantly improved my overall wellbeing, making me feel more vibrant and productive throughout the day. It is something I will maintain at least a few days each fortnight.

Directions for use:

- If you don't have a juicer yet, get one!
- Buy fresh celery, ideally organic.
- Wash it in a sink with baking soda and white or apple cider vinegar.
- Juice enough celery to make about 600 ml.
- Drink it right away for the best results.
- Consume in the morning on an empty stomach for optimal absorption.

Sauna

Research by Dr Jari Laukkanen from the University of Eastern Finland suggests that regular *sauna use could cut the risk of severe mental health issues by up to 80%.* Saunas, which heat up to between 150 °F and 195 °F (65 °C to 90 °C), offer a cosy space that can be dry or steamy, depending on the type.

Saunas are traditionally used for relaxation and to promote sweating, which can have various health benefits. Dr Joy Hussain from RMIT University reviewed 40 clinical studies and found that saunas can greatly improve your mood and reduce mental health symptoms.

Directions for use:

- Make sure you're well-hydrated.
- Wear light clothing.
- Start with 10–15-minute sessions if you're new to it.
- Gradually extend to 15–20 minutes as you get used to the heat.
- Avoid staying in for more than 45 minutes total.
- If you start feeling dizzy or uncomfortable, step out and rehydrate.

Cold water therapy

Cold water therapy might actually work better than antidepressant medications for some people. A review of 10 studies led by Julia Doets from the Mental Health Service Organization in Europe found that plunging into cold water led to big improvements in mental health, especially for depression.

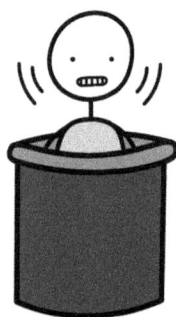

I'm a huge advocate for this approach. It makes an overwhelming difference in my life—it's as useful as a morning coffee for me!

Cold water therapy, also called hydrotherapy or cold water immersion, involves soaking your body in cold water. This can boost levels of norepinephrine and beta-endorphins in your blood, which can help improve your mood.

Research varies on how long cold exposure should be for mental health benefits. Dr Nikolai Shevchuk from Virginia Commonwealth University found that just 2 to 3 minutes can help, while Didrik Espeland's research at the Arctic University of Norway suggests around 10 minutes to see a big improvement in symptoms.

Directions for use:

- Always pay attention to how your body feels.
- Talk to a healthcare professional if you have any medical conditions before you start.
- Begin slowly and carefully to avoid risks like hypothermia or shock.
- Start by turning off the warm water for the last few seconds of your shower.
- Gradually increase the time as you get used to the cold, aiming for 4 to 10 minutes.
- Keep the water temperature between 50–59 °F (10–15 °C).
- Choose whatever works best for you, whether that's cold showers, baths, or even a dip in the ocean with a cold water swimming club.
- Try cold water therapy daily or at least once a week.

Massage

Massage therapy is a hands-on treatment that involves pressing, rubbing, and manipulating muscles, tendons, ligaments, and skin to help relax the body, reduce pain, and boost overall health. There are different types of massage, such as Swedish, deep tissue, sports, and trigger point, each tailored to specific needs.

This therapy not only helps to ease muscle tension and improve circulation but also reduces stress and anxiety and boosts the immune system. Recent research by Dr Christopher Moyer from the University of Illinois Urbana-Champaign, which examined 37 independent studies, found that massage therapy significantly reduces symptoms of common mental health concerns, enhancing both physical and mental wellbeing.

Directions for use:

- Try to schedule regular sessions, ideally once a week or every 2 weeks.

- Choose a type of massage that best fits your needs: Swedish massage is great for relaxation and stress relief, while deep tissue or trigger point massage is better for easing muscle tension.
- Make sure to find a licensed and experienced massage therapist who can customise the massage to address your specific mental health needs.

Light therapy

Light therapy, or phototherapy, involves sitting near a lightbox that mimics natural sunlight. It's mostly used to treat seasonal affective disorder, a type of depression that usually occurs in the winter, but it can also help with other conditions, promote general mental health, and regulate sleep patterns.

For example, a review of 8 studies by Dr Robert Golden from the University of North Carolina found that light therapy can significantly reduce mental health symptoms by regulating sleep and increasing serotonin levels in the brain. His 2023 study also showed that regular light therapy sessions improve mood, energy, and overall mental wellbeing, making it a helpful treatment for a variety of mental health conditions.

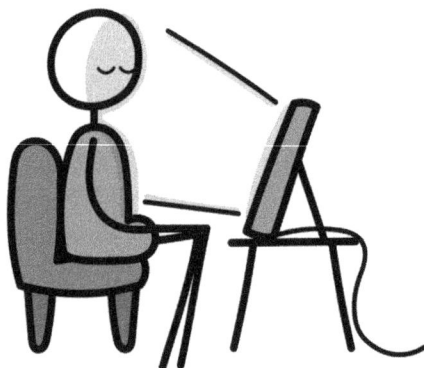

Direction for use:

- Choose a light box that emits at least 10,000 lux of light and filters out ultraviolet (UV) rays.

- Use light therapy in the morning, right after you wake up to help regulate your sleep cycle and boost your mood for the day.

- Avoid using it in the afternoon or evening, as it can interfere with your sleep.

- Start with just a few minutes per session and gradually work up to 20 to 30 minutes a day.

- Place the light box at eye level, about 40 to 60 cm away from where you are sitting.

- Keep your eyes open, but don't look directly at the light. You can go about your usual morning routine, such as eating breakfast or reading, during the session.

- Some people might experience mild side effects at first, such as headaches, eye strain, or nausea, but these typically go away over time or with adjustments to the duration or intensity of light exposure.

Forest bathing

Forest bathing, or *Shinrin-yoku*, is a Japanese practice where you immerse yourself in a forest or natural setting and mindfully take in your surroundings to boost both mental and physical health. This concept, which started in Japan in the 1980s, has become a popular holistic wellness activity. The idea is to engage all your senses and connect deeply with nature.

A recent review by Dr Margaret Hansen from the University of San Francisco examined 64 studies to evaluate the effects of spending time in forest environments. The findings show that forest bathing can significantly lower cortisol levels and reduce stress, anxiety, and depression, while also improving mood and overall psychological wellbeing. This might be partly due to phytoncides, natural chemicals released by trees, which can enhance neurotransmitter production when inhaled. Forest bathing is part of a growing recognition of nature's therapeutic benefits for mental health.

Directions for use:

- Pick a peaceful spot with lots of natural surroundings, such as a forest with no roads or trails.
- Spend at least 2 hours there.
- Leave your phone and other devices behind so that you can stay focused.
- Use all your senses: look at the colours around you, listen to the birds and rustling leaves, breathe in the fresh forest air, and feel the texture of tree bark and leaves.
- Aim to do this once a week or more for the best experience.

Grounding

I've only recently starting this practice. I combine it with my lemon water and morning sun as a form of habit stacking. I do seem to feel more relaxed following a session.

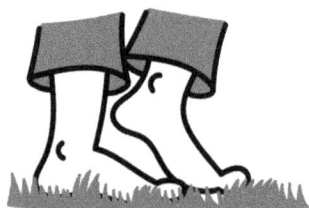

Grounding, or earthing, is a technique that helps you reconnect with the Earth's natural energy. It involves accessing the Earth's natural electrons via activities such as walking barefoot on grass or sand, lying on the ground, or using grounding gear indoors.

Dr Gaétan Chevalier from the University of California recently reviewed studies on grounding and found it can help reduce stress, mental health issues, and fatigue. It also improves mood, psychological wellbeing, and sleep, making it a simple and affordable way to boost mental health.

Directions for use:

- Try walking barefoot on grass, sand, or soil or simply lie on the ground.
- Aim for 20 to 30 minutes each day.

- You can also swim in natural bodies of water such as oceans, lakes, or rivers.
- If you prefer staying indoors, you can use grounding mats, sheets, or bands that plug into a grounded outlet. There are even shoes with conductive soles for grounding.
- Aim to ground daily.

Hydrogen water

Hydrogen water, or hydrogen-rich water, is regular water that's been infused with hydrogen gas. This hydrogen acts as a powerful antioxidant, helping to neutralise harmful molecules which damage your cells (free radicals) in your body. A review by Dr Shigeo Ohta from Nippon Medical School found that hydrogen water can reduce oxidative stress and inflammation, which are linked to mental health issues. It may also boost brain function and improve mood by tackling oxidative damage (caused by free radicals) and inflammation.

Directions for use:

- Pick reputable brands that guarantee a good amount of dissolved hydrogen.
- You can also use a hydrogen water generator or tablets to infuse water yourself.
- Try drinking hydrogen water 1 to 3 times a day.
- Start with a small amount to see how you feel, then gradually increase if needed.
- Drink it on an empty stomach, such as first thing in the morning or between meals.
- Keep hydrogen water in a sealed container to keep the hydrogen from escaping and drink it soon after opening to get the most benefit.

Spore-based probiotic

You've probably tried probiotics such as Yakult or kombucha before, but some research suggests that many of these might not survive your stomach acid long enough to help your gut.

Doctor Ami Sperber led a 73,000-person global study out of Ben-Gurion University and found that nearly 40% of adults have gut issues. That's where probiotics come in—often advertised as a cure-all.

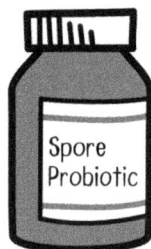

But there's another type called spore-based probiotics. These contain bacterial spores that are really tough and can survive the stomach's acidity. Once they reach your intestines, they activate and start working to improve your gut health. Common examples are *Bacillus coagulans*, *Bacillus subtilis*, and *Bacillus clausii*. Research led by Natasha Williams at Colorado State University suggests these spore-based probiotics, especially *B. subtilis*, might be the most effective for gut health.

Directions for use:

- Choose a spore-based probiotic (the label will say this).
- If you can, pick one with all 3 strains: B. coagulans, B. subtilis, and B. clausii.
- Follow the dosage on the label, usually 1 to 5 billion colony-forming units a day.
- Take it with a meal.
- Use it daily for 3 months, then take a break for 3 months.

Filtered water

Filtered water is water that's been cleaned using different methods to get rid of impurities and harmful substances. This can include using activated carbon filters, reverse osmosis, ceramic filters, or UV light. These methods can remove things like fluoride, chlorine, bacteria, and heavy metals, which can negatively affect mental health.

In a 24,000-person study led by Dr Shuduo Zhou at Peking University, researchers looked at how metals and other elements in drinking water might impact mental health. They found that drinking unfiltered water containing these elements was linked to more mental health issues.

Directions for use:

- Pick a water filter that suits your needs, such as activated carbon filters, reverse osmosis systems, or UV light purifiers.
- Try to drink about 8 glasses, or 2 litres, of filtered water each day to stay hydrated.
- You might need more or less depending on your activity and surroundings.
- Make sure to keep your filter in good shape by following the manufacturer's instructions for maintenance and replacement.
- When you're travelling or in places where clean water might be hard to find, use portable water filters or filtered water in bottles.

Complementary approaches take-home message

These extra approaches are like bonus tools you can use alongside the main steps in this guide to boost your mental health. They include different practices that are showing real promise for improving mental wellbeing in various ways. Think of them as helpful extras for managing symptoms or staying symptom-free.

Congratulations!

Well done on working through this guide and learning how to create excellent mental health!

Remember, looking after your mental health is a journey that needs ongoing effort. It's about being aware of your needs, having the courage to try new strategies, and staying dedicated to what works for you. We've covered a lot of different ways to support your mental wellbeing, and now you have a toolkit you can use whenever you need to.

One big takeaway is the importance of a holistic approach to mental health. This means understanding that your mind and body are connected and affect each other. For example, getting screened for any underlying health issues or nutrient deficiencies can help you pinpoint what might be impacting how you feel. Supplements might be needed to give your body the extra support it needs. Getting enough sleep, eating well, and staying active all play a huge role in boosting your mood. Staying socially connected is also incredibly important for your mental wellbeing. Taking time for self-care and hobbies, reducing your screen time, and practising CBT techniques can also help you manage and improve your mental health.

It's important to remember that there's no one-size-fits-all solution for mental health. What works for one person might not work for another. Be open to experimenting with different strategies, listen to your mind and body, and be patient with yourself.

The steps in this guide can be used not just to manage current symptoms, but also to help prevent future issues. And while this guide provides tools to help you manage things on your own, remember that seeking professional help when you need it is a sign of strength, not weakness.

Ultimately, the goal is to build a resilient and meaningful life in which your mental health is a priority. Embrace the practices that make you feel your best and remember that taking care of your mental health is a continuous, evolving process. Celebrate your progress, no matter how small, and know that by prioritising your mental health, you are investing in a happier, healthier future.

Acknowledgements

To my readers, thank you for embarking on this journey of self-discovery with me. Your courage and commitment to improving your mental health are the heart of this guide.

I am deeply indebted to those close to me for their steadfast support and unwavering encouragement throughout this journey. Your love, guidance and understanding have been an encouragement guiding me through the challenges and triumphs of writing this guide.

I am deeply grateful to all those who supported and guided me in the creation of this guide. Your staunch encouragement and love have been my foundation.

Special thanks to my editors, Merridy Pugh, Dr Liz Charpleix and Amara Motala, and my cover designer and illustrator, Kylie Dunn, whose insightful feedback, creativity and expertise were invaluable.

To the mental health professionals and researchers whose work inspired many of these pages, your dedication is truly admirable.

Lastly, I extend genuine gratitude to the world-leading researchers and educators whose tireless dedication informed my path towards greater comprehension and compassionate mental health care. Your wisdom, guidance, and unwavering commitment to advancing knowledge have profoundly shaped and inspired me and this work.

About the Author

Colby is a registered psychologist with a wide range of experience. He's worked in various settings, including child protection, emergency suicide and crisis support, clinical psychology, behaviour support, a national sports team, and a leading university research team. His education in psychology is extensive—he's earned a Bachelor of Psychological Science, a Graduate Diploma of Psychology, and a Master of Applied Psychology. His outstanding performance during his master's degree earned him life membership in the Golden Key International Honor Society.

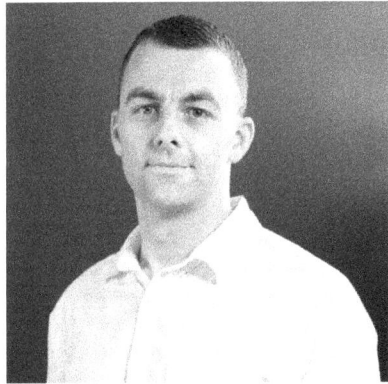

In addition to his degrees, Colby has completed training in applied suicide intervention skills and mental health first aid. Before diving into psychology, he studied health science, focusing on nutrition, health promotion, and physical activity and health, which shaped his holistic approach to mental health.

Colby has published several research articles in international, peer-reviewed journals, covering topics including mental health, substance use, nutritional support, physical activity interventions, and empowerment. He has collaborated with renowned academics in Australia on these projects. Recently, Colby was honoured with the Victorian University Rising Star Alumni Award for his dedication to mental health research and practice.

Now based in Melbourne, Victoria, Colby grew up in the small country town of Warracknabeal. He loves being outdoors and staying active and has a strong passion for nutrition and looking at mental health through a holistic lens.

Research Overview

Introduction

Noam Shpancer
Shpancer, N. (2012). *The good psychologist.* **Oxford University Press.** This book, authored by Noam Shpancer, provided the following quote "Mental health is not a destination, but a process. It's about how you drive, not where you're going."

Understanding Mental Health

George L. Engel
Engel, G. L. (1977). The need for a new medical model: a challenge for biomedicine. *Science, 196*(4286), 129-136. This research, authored by George L. Engel from the University of Rochester School of Medicine, advocates for a biopsychosocial

model, which offers a comprehensive framework for research, teaching, and practical application in healthcare.

William Lugg

Lugg, W. (2022). The biopsychosocial model–history, controversy and Engel. *Australasian Psychiatry*, *30*(1), 55- **59.** This research, authored by William Lugg from the Royal Prince Alfred Hospital, reviewed the history and development of the biopsychosocial (BPS) model, emphasising its lasting relevance in psychiatry. Despite criticism, the BPS model, introduced in the 1940s and expanded by George Engel in 1977, integrates psychological, biological, and sociocultural factors to better understand mental disorders.

World Health Organization

World Health Organization. (2022) Mental disorders. World Health Organization. www.who.int/news- room/fact-sheets/detail/mental-disorders This article from the World Health Organization reports that 1 in 8 people globally live with a mental disorder, impacting thinking, emotions, and behaviour. Despite available treatments, most lack access to care. Conditions include anxiety, depression, and schizophrenia. Stigma and resource shortages persist, highlighting the need for comprehensive global mental health strategies.

Symptom Checklist

American Psychiatric Association

American Psychiatric Association. (2013). *Diagnostic and statistical manual of mental disorders* **(5th ed.). American Psychiatric Association.** This book, authored by the American Psychiatric Association, provides criteria for diagnosing mental disorders, incorporating the latest research and clinical findings to guide mental health professionals in identifying, classifying, and understanding various psychiatric conditions.

Matt Haig

Haig, M. (2015). *Reasons to stay alive.* **Canongate Books.**
This book authored by Matt Haig, explores his own personal battle with depression and anxiety. Through heartfelt reflections, Haig offers insights on mental health, the challenges of recovery, and the importance of hope, resilience, and human connection in overcoming life's darkest moments.

Step One: Health Screening

Şerife Akpınar

Akpınar, Ş., & Karadağ, M. G. (2022). Is vitamin D important in anxiety or depression? What is the truth? *Current Nutrition Reports, 11*(4), 675-681. This research, led by Şerife Akpınar from Gazi University, examined the link between vitamin D and mood disorders, such as depression and anxiety. It investigated how oxidative stress and inflammation relate to these disorders and vitamin D metabolism. Findings suggest that low vitamin D is linked to increased symptoms, emphasising the importance of monitoring levels for prevention and treatment.

Dr Ali Alzahrani

Alzahrani, A. S., Al Mourad, M., Hafez, K., Almaghamsy, A. M., Alamri, F. A., Al Juhani, N. R., ... & Abdelhamid, E. (2020). Diagnosis and management of hypothyroidism in Gulf Cooperation Council (GCC) countries. *Advances in Therapy, 37*(7), 3097-3111. This research, led by Dr Ali Alzahrani from King Faisal Specialist Hospital and Research Centre, assessed hypothyroidism diagnosis and management in Saudi Arabia and the GCC. Led by Saudi endocrinologists, it reviewed current practices and made recommendations, emphasising the importance of screening high-risk groups and addressing the condition's broader impact.

Professor Regan Bailey

Bailey, R. L., Carmel, R., Green, R., Pfeiffer, C. M.,

Cogswell, M. E., Osterloh, J. D., ... & Yetley, E. A. (2011). **Monitoring of vitamin B-12 nutritional status in the United States by using plasma methylmalonic acid and serum vitamin B-12.** *The American Journal of Clinical Nutrition, 94*(2), 552-561. This research, led by Professor Regan Bailey from the National Institutes of Health, analysed data from 12,612 US adults to assess how different cutoffs for vitamin B12 affect deficiency rates. The study found that varying thresholds, particularly using a cutoff of >148 pmol/L for B12, led to misclassifications. These findings emphasise the need for consistent diagnostic standards.

Ansley Bender
Bender, A., Hagan, K. E., & Kingston, N. (2017). The association of folate and depression: A meta-analysis. *Journal of Psychiatric Research, 95*, 9-18. This research, led by Ansley Bender from the University of South Florida, undertook a meta-analysis of 28 studies comparing folate levels in individuals with and without depression. The findings revealed that those with depression had notably lower folate levels (Hedge's g = −0.24), suggesting a small but significant effect.

Dr Will Cole
Cole, W. (2024, January 23). Do you have the gene mutation that affects 40% of the world? Dr. Will Cole. **https://drwillcole.com/brain-health/do-you-have-the-gene-mutation-that-affects-40-of-the-world** This article, authored by Dr Will Cole, explores the prevalence and impact of the *MTHFR* gene mutation, affecting up to 40% of the global population. It explains how this genetic variation can influence brain function and overall wellness and underscores the importance of genetic testing and personalised treatment approaches for managing the mutation's health effects.

Aiyong Cui
Cui, A., Zhang, T., Xiao, P., Fan, Z., Wang, H., & Zhuang, Y. (2023). Global and regional prevalence of vitamin D deficiency in population-based studies from

2000 to 2022: A pooled analysis of 7.9 million participants. *Frontiers in Nutrition, 10,* **1070808.** This research, led by Aiyong Cui from Xi'an Jiaotong University, undertook a meta-analysis of 308 studies, involving 7,947,359 participants from 81 countries, to assess global and regional vitamin D deficiency between 2000 and 2022. It found that 15.7% of people had serum vitamin D levels below 30 nmol/L, with higher deficiency rates in high-latitude regions, especially during winter and spring.

Ewelina Dziurkowska
Dziurkowska, E., & Wesolowski, M. (2021). Cortisol as a biomarker of mental disorder severity. *Journal of Clinical Medicine, 10*(21), **5204.** This research, led by Ewelina Dziurkowska from the Medical University of Gdansk, reviewed how cortisol, a key hormone affecting metabolism and the central nervous system, could serve as a biological marker for mental illness. It examined cortisol fluctuations in psychiatric disorders such as depression, bipolar disorder, and psychosis, and evaluated the impact of therapies and medications on cortisol levels.

Dr Charles Gant
Integrative Psychotherapy Omaha. (2014). Functional medicine for mental health. Integrative Psychotherapy Omaha. https://integrativepsychotherapyomaha.com/functional-medicine-for-mental-health/ This article features insights from Dr Charles Gant, explaining how functional medicine can address mental health issues. It highlights the benefits of a holistic approach, including personalised treatments and comprehensive assessments, which aim to improve mental wellbeing by targeting underlying physiological imbalances and lifestyle factors.

Eamon Laird
Laird, E. J., O'Halloran, A. M., Molloy, A. M., Healy, M., Hernandez, B., O'Connor, D. M., ... & Briggs, R. (2021). Low vitamin B12 but not folate is associated with incident

depressive symptoms in community-dwelling older adults: A 4-year longitudinal study. *British Journal of Nutrition, 130*(2), 268-275. This research, led by Eamon Laird from the University of Limerick, followed 3,849 adults aged 50 and over for 4 years, exploring the connection between blood levels of folate and B12 and the development of depression. It found that low B12 levels increased the risk of depression by 51%, while folate levels had no significant impact.

Dr Rogers
Rogers, L. M., Cordero, A. M., Pfeiffer, C. M., Hausman, D. B., Tsang, B. L., De-Regil, L. M., ... & Bailey, L. B. (2018). Global folate status in women of reproductive age: A systematic review with emphasis on methodological issues. *Annals of the New York Academy of Sciences, 1431*(1), 35-57. This research, led by Dr Rogers from the World Health Organization, reviewed data from 45 surveys across 39 countries to assess folate levels in women of reproductive age. It found that over 20% of women in lower-income countries were folate deficient, compared to less than 5% in higher-income nations. Folate insufficiency was widespread, affecting over 40% in many areas.

Dr Nader Salari
Salari, N., Hosseinian-Far, A., Jalali, R., Vaisi-Raygani, A., Rasoulpoor, S., Mohammadi, M., ... & Khaledi-Paveh, B. (2020). Prevalence of stress, anxiety, depression among the general population during the COVID-19 pandemic: A systematic review and meta-analysis. *Globalization and Health, 16*, 1-11. This research, led by Dr Nader Salari from Kermanshah University of Medical Sciences, looked at 36 studies with over 113,000 participants to explore the impact of the COVID-19 pandemic on mental health. The findings showed that 29.6% of people experienced stress, 31.9% dealt with anxiety, and 33.7% faced depression.

Tan Yongjun
Tan, Y., Zhou, L., Gu, K., Xie, C., Wang, Y., Cha, L., ... &

Yang, Q. (2023). Correlation between vitamin B12 and mental health in children and adolescents: A systematic review and meta-analysis. *Clinical Psychopharmacology and Neuroscience, 21*(4), 617-633. This research, led by Tan Yongjun from the Hospital of Chongqing Medical University, analysed 56 studies involving nearly 38,000 participants to investigate the link between vitamin B12 and mental health. The findings revealed that those with higher vitamin B12 intakes had a reduced risk of depression and behavioural issues.

Step Two: Targeted Supplementation

Jaqueline Borges-Vieira and Camila Souza Cardoso
Borges-Vieira, J. G., & Cardoso, C. K. S. (2023). Efficacy of B vitamins and vitamin D therapy in improving depressive and anxiety disorders: A systematic review of randomized controlled trials. *Nutritional Neuroscience, 26*(3), 187-207. This research, led by Jaqueline Borges-Vieira from the Catholic University of Goiás in Brazil, evaluated 20 randomised controlled trials involving over 2,200 participants to look at the effects of B vitamins and vitamin D on depression and anxiety disorders. The findings showed that taking folic acid, B1, B12, and vitamin D significantly lowered depression scores and enhanced standard treatments. However, the evidence for anxiety improvement was mainly linked to vitamin D.

Dr Neil Boyle
Boyle, N. B., Lawton, C., & Dye, L. (2017). The effects of magnesium supplementation on subjective anxiety and stress—A systematic review. *Nutrients, 9*(5), 429. This research, led by Dr Neil Boyle from the University of Leeds, looked at 18 studies on magnesium (Mg) supplementation for anxiety, focusing on individuals with existing anxiety vulnerabilities. The findings suggested that magnesium might be helpful for some groups, such as those with premenstrual syndrome or mild anxiety.

Dr Gleicilaine Casseb

Casseb, G. A., Kaster, M. P., & Rodrigues, A. L. S. (2019). Potential role of vitamin D for the management of depression and anxiety. *CNS Drugs*, *33*(7), 619-637. This research, led by Dr Gleicilaine Casseb from the Center for Biological Sciences in Brazil, examined both preclinical and clinical evidence on vitamin D supplementation for major depressive disorder (MDD) and anxiety. Out of 13 studies on MDD, 12 reported positive results. While vitamin D appears to be beneficial, the variation in outcomes suggests that more research is needed to understand factors like initial vitamin D levels, supplementation methods, and individual differences.

Fatemeh Fadaki

Fadaki, F., Modaresi, M., & Sajjadian, I. (2017). The effects of ginger extract and diazepam on anxiety reduction in animal model. *Indian Journal of Pharmaceutical Education and Research*, *51*(3), S159-S162. This research, led by Fatemeh Fadaki from Islamic Azad University, used 60 female mice to investigate the effects of ginger extract and diazepam on anxiety. The mice were divided into different groups, including a control group, an anxiety group, a diazepam group, and 3 groups receiving varying doses of ginger extract (50, 100, and 200 mg/kg). The results showed that ginger extract significantly reduced anxiety and increased movement activity at the 200 mg/kg dose, suggesting it might be a viable alternative to diazepam.

Dr Laura Fusar-Poli

Fusar-Poli, L., Vozza, L., Gabbiadini, A., Vanella, A., Concas, I., Tinacci, S., ... & Aguglia, E. (2020). Curcumin for depression: A meta-analysis. *Critical Reviews in Food Science and Nutrition*, *60*(15), 2643-2653. This research, led by Dr Laura Fusar-Poli from the University of Catania, reviewed 9 studies with 531 participants to examine curcumin's effects on depression and anxiety. The findings indicated that curcumin led to significant improvements in both depressive symptoms

(Hedge's g = −0.75) and anxiety symptoms (Hedge's g = −2.62), demonstrating large effect sizes. These results suggest that curcumin may enhance standard care for these conditions.

Yuhua Liao

Liao, Y., Xie, B., Zhang, H., He, Q., Guo, L., Subramanieapillai, M., ... & McIntyre, R. S. (2019). Efficacy of omega-3 PUFAs in depression: A meta-analysis. *Translational Psychiatry*, *9*(1), 190. This research, led by Yuhua Liao from the Chinese Center for Chronic Disease Control, reviewed 26 double-blind randomised controlled trials involving 2,160 participants to investigate the effects of omega-3 polyunsaturated fatty acids (PUFAs), specifically EPA and DHA, on depression. The analysis found a significant overall benefit (standardised mean difference = −0.28, P = 0.004). Notably, EPA formulations containing at least 60% EPA at doses of 1 gram per day showed clinical benefits.

Dr Yu-Fang Lin

Lin, Y. F., Zhu, J. F., Chen, Y. D., Sheng, J. L., He, J. J., Zhang, S. Y., & Jin, X. Q. (2020). Effect of ginger separated moxibustion on fatigue, sleep quality and depression in patients with chronic fatigue syndrome: A randomized controlled trial. *Zhongguo Zhen jiu= Chinese Acupuncture & Moxibustion*, *40*(8), 816-820. This research led by Dr Yu-Fang Lin from the Department of Acupuncture and Moxibustion at Zhejiang Hospital in China involved 62 participants to evaluate the effects of ginger-separated moxibustion on fatigue, sleep quality, and depression in patients with chronic fatigue syndrome. The ginger group experienced significant improvements in all areas compared to the non-ginger group. Measurements using the Short Form Health Survey (SF-36), Pittsburgh Sleep Quality Index, and Self-Rating Depression Scale all showed better results in the ginger group after treatment (P < 0.01).

Professor Robert McNamara

McNamara, R. K. (2016). Role of omega-3 fatty acids in the etiology, treatment, and prevention of depression: Current status and future directions. *Journal of Nutrition & Intermediary Metabolism, 5*, 96-106. This research, led by Professor Robert McNamara from the University of Cincinnati, examined the link between long-chain omega-3 (LCn-3) fatty acid deficiency, including EPA and DHA, and major depressive disorder (MDD). It highlighted that MDD patients often have lower levels of EPA and DHA in their red blood cells. The review discussed the potential antidepressant effects of EPA/DHA supplementation. It suggests that dietary LCn-3 deficiency could be a modifiable risk factor for MDD.

Mahdi Moabedi

Moabedi, M., Aliakbari, M., Erfanian, S., & Milajerdi, A. (2023). Magnesium supplementation beneficially affects depression in adults with depressive disorder: A systematic review and meta-analysis of randomized clinical trials. *Frontiers in Psychiatry, 14*, 1333261. This research, led by Mahdi Moabedi from Kashan University of Medical Sciences, reviewed 7 randomised clinical trials with 325 participants to investigate the effects of magnesium supplementation on depression. The findings revealed a significant reduction in depression scores with magnesium (standardised mean difference: −0.919, 95% Confidence Interval: −1.443 to −0.396, P = 0.001). The review suggests that magnesium supplementation may be beneficial for those experiencing depression.

Dr Bettina Moritz

Moritz, B., Schmitz, A. E., Rodrigues, A. L. S., Dafre, A. L., & Cunha, M. P. (2020). The role of vitamin C in stress-related disorders. *The Journal of Nutritional Biochemistry, 85*, 108459. This research, led by Dr Bettina Moritz from the Federal University of Santa Catarina, explored the potential of ascorbic acid (vitamin C) as a treatment for stress-related disorders, including depression and anxiety. It summarised the biological functions of vitamin C and its role in maintaining central nervous system (CNS) balance, while reviewing studies on its effects. The evidence suggests that vitamin C supplementation can enhance mood and has antidepressant effects, all with low toxicity.

Dr Uma Naidoo

Naidoo, U. (2021). *This is your brain on food: An illustrated guide to the surprising foods that help us think, feel, and thrive*. **Little, Brown Spark.** This book, authored by Dr Uma Naidoo, examines the link between diet and mental health. It provides insights into how different foods and nutrients, especially B vitamins, influence brain function, mood, and overall wellbeing. The book also offers practical advice on improving mental health through nutrition.

Somave Yosaee

Yosaee, S., Clark, C. C., Keshtkaran, Z., Ashourpour, M., Keshani, P., & Soltani, S. (2022). **Zinc in depression: From development to treatment: A comparative/dose response meta-analysis of observational studies and randomized controlled trials.** *General Hospital Psychiatry*, **74**, 110-117. This research, led by doctoral candidate Somave Yosaee from Larestan University of Medical Sciences, reviewed data from randomised controlled trials and observational studies involving 1,264 participants to assess the impact of zinc on depression. The findings showed that zinc supplementation significantly reduced depressive symptoms and lowered the risk of depression by 28%, particularly when used on its own.

Step Three: Sleep

Dr Arman Arab

Arab, A., Rafie, N., Amani, R., & Shirani, F. (2023). **The role of magnesium in sleep health: A systematic review of available literature.** *Biological Trace Element Research,*

201(1), 121-128. This research, led by Dr Arman Arab from Isfahan University of Medical Sciences, examined 9 studies involving 7,582 adults to explore the relationship between magnesium (Mg) and sleep quality. The observational studies indicated a positive association between magnesium levels and improved sleep quality.

Fiona Auld

Auld, F., Maschauer, E. L., Morrison, I., Skene, D. J., & Riha, R. L. (2017). Evidence for the efficacy of melatonin in the treatment of primary adult sleep disorders. *Sleep Medicine Reviews,* **34, 10-22.** This research, led by Fiona Auld from the Department of Sleep Medicine at the Royal Infirmary Edinburgh, reviewed 12 randomised controlled trials involving 5,030 participants to assess the effectiveness of exogenous melatonin for treating primary sleep disorders. The findings indicated that melatonin significantly reduced the time it took to fall asleep in cases of primary insomnia and delayed sleep phase syndrome, and it helped regulate sleep–wake patterns.

Professor Oliviero Bruni

Bruni, O., Ferini-Strambi, L., Giacomoni, E., & Pellegrino, P. (2021). Herbal remedies and their possible effect on the GABAergic system and sleep. *Nutrients,* **13(2), 530.** This research, led by Professor Oliviero Bruni from Sapienza University, reviews herbal treatments for insomnia, including valerian, passionflower, and lavender, which are well-regarded for their safety and effectiveness. The findings suggest that these herbs may reduce the time it takes to fall asleep and enhance sleep quality by interacting with GABA receptors and modulating GABAergic signalling.

Amanda Bulman

Bulman, A., D'Cunha, N., Marx, W., Turner, M., McKune, A., & Naumovski, N. (2023). The effects of l-theanine supplementation on quality of sleep: A systematic review. *Proceedings,* **91(1), 32.** This research, led by Amanda Bulman from the University of Canberra, evaluated the effects of L-theanine (L-THE) on sleep quality by analysing 11 studies with 373 adults and 107 children. The findings indicated that L-theanine, at doses ranging from 50 to 655 mg, improved several sleep parameters, including the time it took to fall asleep and overall sleep quality. However, doses exceeding 655 mg may have the opposite effect.

Dr Zachary Caddick
Caddick, Z. A., Gregory, K., Arsintescu, L., & Flynn-Evans, E. E. (2018). A review of the environmental parameters necessary for an optimal sleep environment. *Building and Environment, 132,* **11-20.** This research, led by Dr Zachary Caddick from the San Jose State Research Foundation, explored the characteristics of an optimal sleep environment. It recommends keeping noise levels below 35 dB, maintaining a temperature between 17–28 °C with 40%–60% humidity, ensuring complete darkness, and avoiding blue light. Ideal conditions include sea-level air quality with good ventilation; supplemental oxygen can improve sleep at higher altitudes.

Dr Colleen Lance
Cleveland Clinic. (2023). What time should I go to bed? Cleveland Clinic. https://health.clevelandclinic.org/what-time-should-i-go-to-bed This article, featuring insights from Dr Colleen Lance, explains that the optimal bedtime depends on individual schedules and sleep needs, but consistency is crucial. It recommends aligning your sleep pattern with your circadian rhythm and highlights that good sleep hygiene, including a regular routine, is essential for maintaining overall health and wellbeing.

Dr Sophie Faulkner
Faulkner, S., & Bee, P. (2016). Perspectives on sleep, sleep problems, and their treatment, in people with serious mental illnesses: A systematic review. *PLoS One, 11*(9), **e0163486.** This research led by Dr Sophie Faulkner from the University of Manchester reviewed 2,067 studies and identified

only 22 relevant papers, focusing on individuals with serious mental illness who often experience sleep issues that impact their functioning and wellbeing. The findings highlight a strong connection between sleep and mental health.

Dr Max Hirshkowitz
Hirshkowitz, M., Whiton, K., Albert, S. M., Alessi, C., Bruni, O., DonCarlos, L., ... & Hillard, P. J. A. (2015). National Sleep Foundation's sleep time duration recommendations: Methodology and results summary. *Sleep Health*, *1*(1), 40-43. This research, led by Dr Max Hirshkowitz from Stanford University, involved an expert panel that updated the National Sleep Foundation's sleep duration recommendations. It suggests that adults need around 7–9 hours of sleep. These guidelines are meant for healthy individuals; any deviations may signal potential health issues.

Dr Andrew Huberman
Huberman, A. (n.d). Myo-inositol for sleep. Huberman Lab. https://ai.hubermanlab.com/clip?sids=chunk_49471 &sids=chunk_49520&sids=chunk_57320 This article from Dr Andrew Huberman explores the benefits of myo-inositol for improving sleep. It explains that myo-inositol, a vitamin-like substance, can enhance sleep quality and help with insomnia by influencing neurotransmitter systems and hormonal balance. This makes it a natural option for promoting restful sleep.

Daniel Kramer
Kramer, D. J., & Johnson, A. A. (2024). Apigenin: A natural molecule at the intersection of sleep and aging. *Frontiers in Nutrition*, *11*, 1359176. This research, led by Daniel Kramer from Tally Health in New York, highlights that Nicotinamide Adenine Dinucleotide (NAD+) is a vital coenzyme found in all living cells, with levels declining as we age. It notes that apigenin, a flavonoid found in chamomile, can boost NAD+ by inhibiting the CD38 enzyme. In animal studies, apigenin has been shown to improve sleep, cognition, and longevity, and it may help reduce cancer growth and

extend lifespan. Human studies suggest that dietary apigenin enhances sleep quality, likely by interacting with GABA and inflammatory pathways.

Dr Oscar Lederman
Lederman, O., Ward, P. B., Firth, J., Maloney, C., Carney, R., Vancampfort, D., … & Rosenbaum, S. (2019). Does exercise improve sleep quality in individuals with mental illness? A systematic review and meta-analysis. *Journal of Psychiatric Research, 109,* **96-106.** This research, led by Dr Oscar Lederman from the University of New South Wales, analysed 8 randomised controlled trials involving 1,329 participants and found that exercise significantly improves sleep quality in people with severe mental illness. The study highlights exercise as an effective non-pharmacological treatment for addressing poor sleep in this population.

Dr Nathaniel Watson
Marshall, L. (2022, March). Get morning light, sleep better at night. WebMD. https://www.webmd.com/sleep-disorders/features/morning-light-better-sleep This article features insights from Dr Nathaniel Watson highlighting the importance of morning sunlight for improving sleep quality by regulating the body's circadian rhythm. Exposure to natural light in the morning boosts alertness, helps set the internal clock for better sleep at night, and can alleviate insomnia or sleep disorders resulting from irregular sleep patterns.

Dr Viviana Lo Martire
Martire, V. L., Caruso, D., Palagini, L., Zoccoli, G., & Bastianini, S. (2020). Stress & sleep: A relationship lasting a lifetime. *Neuroscience & Biobehavioral Reviews, 117,* **65-77.** This research, led by Dr Viviana Lo Martire from the University of Bologna, examined how stress affects sleep through the hypothalamic–pituitary–adrenal (HPA) axis. It highlights findings from both human and rodent studies showing that stress disrupts sleep homeostasis, with both acute and chronic stress impacting the wake-sleep cycle. Long-term

effects, including those from perinatal stress, can lead to persistent sleep problems.

Dr Janjira Soh

Soh, J., Raventhiran, S., Lee, J. H., Lim, Z. X., Goh, J., Kennedy, B. K., & Maier, A. B. (2024). The effect of glycine administration on the characteristics of physiological systems in human adults: A systematic review. *GeroScience, 46*(1), 219-239. This research, led by Dr Janjira Soh from the National University Health System, assessed the effects of glycine on 11 physiological systems in adults. It found that glycine offers promising benefits, especially for the nervous system and psychiatric symptoms. Short-term glycine administration was shown to improve sleep in healthy individuals.

Dr Christine Spadola

Spadola, C. E., Guo, N., Johnson, D. A., Sofer, T., Bertisch, S. M., Jackson, C. L., ... & Redline, S. (2019). Evening intake of alcohol, caffeine, and nicotine: Night-to-night associations with sleep duration and continuity among African Americans in the Jackson Heart Sleep Study. *Sleep, 42*(11), zsz136. This research, led by Dr Christine Spadola from Florida Atlantic University, investigated the effects of evening alcohol, caffeine, and nicotine use on sleep in 785 African American adults. It found that using alcohol and nicotine within 4 hours of bedtime was associated with lower sleep efficiency and more fragmented sleep, while caffeine did not show significant effects.

Dr Sofia Triantafillou

Triantafillou, S., Saeb, S., Lattie, E. G., Mohr, D. C., & Kording, K. P. (2019). Relationship between sleep quality and mood: Ecological momentary assessment study. *JMIR Mental Health, 6*(3), e12613. This research, led by Dr Sofia Triantafillou from the University of Pennsylvania, involved 208 adults who used mobile phones to track their daily mood and sleep. The findings showed that sleep quality has a stronger influence on the next day's mood than the other way around. While there was a significant bidirectional relationship, sleep quality was found to have a greater impact on mood. Notably, external factors like stress or weather did not affect these results.

Dr Michael Wainberg
Wainberg, M., Jones, S. E., Beaupre, L. M., Hill, S. L., Felsky, D., Rivas, M. A., … & Tripathy, S. J. (2021). Association of accelerometer-derived sleep measures with lifetime psychiatric diagnoses: A cross-sectional study of 89,205 participants from the UK Biobank. *PLoS Medicine*, *18*(10), e1003782. This research, led by Dr Michael Wainberg from the Centre for Addiction and Mental Health in Canada, involved 89,205 participants from the UK Biobank who wore wrist accelerometers. The findings revealed that sleep patterns are associated with various psychiatric disorders and polygenic risk scores. Differences in sleep quality were noted across different diagnoses, suggesting that sleep measures could be valuable in psychiatric research and practice.

Step Four: Balanced Nutrition

Dr Gasem Abu-Taweel
Abu-Taweel, G. M. (2020). Celery ameliorating against neurobehavioral and neurochemical disorders of perinatal lipopolysaccharides exposure in mice offspring. *Journal of King Saud University-Science*, *32*(2), 1764-1771. This research by Dr Gasem Abu-Taweel from Jazan University investigated the effects of lipopolysaccharides (LPS) on neurochemical and behavioural changes in mouse offspring, exploring celery (Apium graveolens) as a potential treatment. The findings revealed that LPS exposure caused developmental delays, cognitive deficits, and reduced neurotransmitter levels. However, celery supplementation helped mitigate these effects, enhancing cognitive function and counteracting the disruptions caused by LPS.

Han Chen

Chen, H., Cao, Z., Hou, Y., Yang, H., Wang, X., & Xu, C. (2023). The associations of dietary patterns with depressive and anxiety symptoms: A prospective study. *BMC Medicine, 21*(1), 307. This research, led by Han Chen from Hangzhou Normal University, involved 126,819 participants from the UK Biobank and found that dietary patterns high in chocolate, confectionery, and butter, but low in fruits and vegetables, were linked to increased symptoms of depression and anxiety. Specifically, higher levels of this dietary pattern were associated with greater odds of depressive symptoms (up to an odds ratio of 1.17) and anxiety symptoms (up to an odds ratio of 1.21).

Dr Heather Colquhoun

Colquhoun, H. L., Squires, J. E., Kolehmainen, N., Fraser, C., & Grimshaw, J. M. (2017). Methods for designing interventions to change healthcare professionals' behaviour: A systematic review. *Implementation Science, 12,* 1-11. This research, led by Dr Heather Colquhoun from the University of Toronto, analysed 15 studies to identify common methods for designing behaviour change interventions. Key strategies included identifying barriers, linking those barriers to intervention components, applying theoretical frameworks, and engaging end users. Most methods targeted individual healthcare professionals, while fewer addressed changes at the organisational or system level.

Dr Arunkumar Dhailappan

Dhailappan, A., & Samiappan, S. (2022). Impact of diet on neurotransmitters. In S. Rajagopal et al. (eds.), *Role of Nutrients in Neurological Disorders* **(pp. 363-383). Springer Singapore.** This book chapter, led by Dr Arunkumar Dhailappan from SNMV College of Arts and Science, examines the significant impact of diet on brain function, emphasising that food quality, rather than just calorie count, is crucial for regulating the nervous system. It highlights how nutrients affect neurotransmitters like GABA, dopamine, and serotonin, which influence brain activity and overall mental health. Additionally, the chapter discusses how excessive consumption of processed foods can contribute to both physical and mental illnesses.

Putu Novi Arfirsta Dharmayani
Dharmayani, P. N. A., Mishra, G. D., & Mihrshahi, S. (2022). Fruit and vegetable consumption and depression symptoms in young women: Results from 1973 to 1978 cohort of the Australian Longitudinal Study on Women's Health. *European Journal of Nutrition*, *61*(8), 4167-4178. This research, led by Putu Novi Arfirsta Dharmayani from Macquarie University, examined the effects of fruit and vegetable consumption on depressive symptoms in 4,241 Australian women over 15 years. The results indicated that higher intake of fruit (4 or more servings) and vegetables (5 or more servings) was consistently linked to lower odds of experiencing depressive symptoms, reducing the risk by 25% and 19%, respectively.

Dr Rubén Fernández-Rodríguez
Fernández-Rodríguez, R., Jiménez-López, E., Garrido-Miguel, M., Martínez-Ortega, I. A., Martínez-Vizcaíno, V., & Mesas, A. E. (2022). Does the evidence support a relationship between higher levels of nut consumption, lower risk of depression, and better mood state in the general population? A systematic review. *Nutrition Reviews*, *80*(10), 2076-2088. This research, led by Dr Rubén Fernández-Rodríguez from Universidad de Castilla-La Mancha, synthesised evidence from 10 studies involving 66,418 individuals to explore the relationship between nut consumption and mental health. The findings suggest that higher nut consumption may be associated with a lower risk of depression and an improved mood.

Celeste Ferraris

Ferraris, C., Scarlett, C. J., Bucher, T., & Beckett, E. L. (2023). **Liking of salt is associated with depression, anxiety, and stress.** *Chemical Senses*, *48*, bjad038. This research, led by Celeste Ferraris from the University of Newcastle, examined 424 Australians and found that a greater preference for salty foods was linked to severe depression and anxiety. Participants with severe depression and anxiety had salt-liking scores of 68.3 and 68.4, respectively, compared to a score of 60.0 in those with normal mood. Moderate stress was also associated with higher salt preference, but only in unadjusted models.

Jeni Fisk

Fisk, J., Khalid, S., Reynolds, S. A., & Williams, C. M. (2020). **Effect of 4 weeks daily wild blueberry supplementation on symptoms of depression in adolescents.** *British Journal of Nutrition*, *124*(2), 181-188. This research, led by Jeni Fisk from the University of Reading, investigated the effects of daily wild blueberry (WBB) supplementation on mood. Over 4 weeks, 64 participants received either WBB or a placebo. The results indicated that those in the WBB group reported significantly fewer symptoms of depression, suggesting potential benefits for preventing depression.

Dr Andrew Saul

Fowler, W. (2017, May). **Do you cashew? Minnesota Good Age.** https://www.mngoodage.com/health/wellness/2017/05/do-you-cashew/ This article features insights from Dr Andrew Saul, exploring the many health benefits of cashews. Rich in healthy fats, protein, and key nutrients like magnesium and zinc, cashews support heart health, strengthen bones, and boost immune function. Including them in a balanced diet can provide a nutritious and health-boosting addition.

Professor Dominika Głąbska

Głąbska, D., Guzek, D., Groele, B., & Gutkowska, K.

(2020). **Fruit and vegetable intake and mental health in adults: A systematic review.** *Nutrients*, *12*(1), 115. This research, led by Professor Dominika Głąbska from Warsaw University of Life Sciences, conducted a systematic review of 61 observational studies examining the association between fruit and vegetable intake and mental health in adults. The findings suggest that higher consumption of fruits and vegetables, particularly berries, citrus, and leafy greens, is linked to better mental health outcomes, including reduced depressive symptoms, less psychological distress, and improved optimism and self-efficacy. Despite variations in study methodologies, the review supports the recommendation to consume at least 5 portions of fruits and vegetables daily for mental health benefits.

Mauritz Herselman

Herselman, M. F., Bailey, S., Deo, P., Zhou, X. F., Gunn, K. M., & Bobrovskaya, L. (2022). The effects of walnuts and academic stress on mental health, general well-being and the gut microbiota in a sample of university students: A randomised clinical trial. *Nutrients*, *14*(22), 4776. This research, led by Mauritz Herselman from the University of South Australia, looked at how academic stress and daily walnut consumption affected university students' mental health and gut health. It found that while academic stress had a negative impact on mood and mental health, eating walnuts daily helped improve mental health and reduced stress-related changes in metabolism and gut microbiota.

Dr Angela Jacques

Jacques, A., Chaaya, N., Beecher, K., Ali, S. A., Belmer, A., & Bartlett, S. (2019). The impact of sugar consumption on stress driven, emotional and addictive behaviours. *Neuroscience & Biobehavioral Reviews*, *103*, 178-199. This research from Dr Angela Jacques from the Queensland University of Technology looked at over 300 studies on how sucrose (sugar) affects the brain, comparing its impact on the mesocorticolimbic system to that of addictive substances. The research shows that sugar can cause changes in brain function and emotional processing, influencing stress, anxiety, and behaviour.

Professor Katherine Keyes
Keyes, K. M., Allel, K., Staudinger, U. M., Ornstein, K. A., & Calvo, E. (2019). Alcohol consumption predicts incidence of depressive episodes across 10 years among older adults in 19 countries. *International Review of Neurobiology, 148,* **1-38.** This research, led by Professor Katherine Keyes from Columbia University, examined 57,276 older adults across 19 countries and found that long-term abstainers and occasional and heavy drinkers were at a higher risk of depressive episodes compared to moderate drinkers. Even after adjusting for other factors, heavy drinking remained strongly linked to depression. Gender and smoking also played a role, with long-term abstainers, women, and smokers showing an increased risk of depression.

Lisa Klevebrant
Klevebrant, L., & Frick, A. (2022). Effects of caffeine on anxiety and panic attacks in patients with panic disorder: A systematic review and meta-analysis. *General Hospital Psychiatry, 74,* **22-31.** This research, led by Lisa Klevebrant from Uppsala University, analysed 10 studies and found that caffeine significantly increased the occurrence of panic attacks in 51.1% of patients with panic disorder (PD), compared to none in the placebo group. It also heightened anxiety in both PD patients and healthy individuals, with PD patients being more sensitive to caffeine's anxiety-inducing effects than healthy controls.

Dr Camille Lassale
Lassale, C., Batty, G. D., Baghdadli, A., Jacka, F., Sanchez-Villegas, A., Kivimaki, M., & Akbaraly, T. (2019). Healthy dietary indices and risk of depressive outcomes: A systematic review and meta-analysis of observational

studies. *Molecular Psychiatry, 24*(7), 965-986. This research, led by Dr Camille Lassale from the University College London, examined 41 studies (20 longitudinal, 21 cross-sectional) on diet quality and depression. It found that high adherence to the Mediterranean diet or a low Dietary Inflammatory Index diet was linked to a reduced risk of depression. The findings suggest that improving diet quality could be a useful strategy for preventing depression.

Dr Edwin McDonald

McDonald, E. (2020). What foods cause or reduce inflammation? UChicago Medicine. https://www. uchicagomedicine.org/forefront/gastrointestinal-articles/what-foods-cause-or-reduce-inflammation This article provides insights from Dr Edwin McDonald, explaining how certain foods can either promote or reduce inflammation in the body. He highlights the benefits of anti-inflammatory foods, such as fruits, vegetables, and healthy fats, in supporting overall health. In contrast, processed foods, sugar, and refined carbohydrates can trigger inflammation and exacerbate health problems.

Dr Uma Naidoo

Naidoo, U. (2022, December 2). Harvard nutritionist and brain expert shares worst foods that weaken memory and focus. CNBC. https://www.cnbc.com/2021/11/28/a-harvard-nutritionist-and-brain-expert-avoids-these-5-foods-that-weaken-memory-and-focus.html This article provides insights from Dr Uma Naidoo, a Harvard nutritionist and brain expert, explaining how certain foods can impair memory and focus. She highlights that processed foods, sugary snacks, fried foods, and refined carbohydrates can cause inflammation, which harms brain function and cognitive health.

Neel Ocean

Ocean, N., Howley, P., & Ensor, J. (2019). Lettuce be happy: A longitudinal UK study on the relationship between fruit and vegetable consumption and well-being.

Social Science & *Medicine*, *222*, 335-345. This research, led by Neel Ocean from the University of Leeds, used UK data from 2010 to 2017 to explore the link between fruit and vegetable consumption and mental wellbeing. The results showed a clear pattern: the more fruits and vegetables people ate, the better their mental wellbeing, even after accounting for other lifestyle factors.

Faezeh Saghafian
Saghafian, F., Malmir, H., Saneei, P., Milajerdi, A., Larijani, B., & Esmaillzadeh, A. (2018). Fruit and vegetable consumption and risk of depression: Accumulative evidence from an updated systematic review and meta-analysis of epidemiological studies. *British Journal of Nutrition*, *119*(10), 1087-1101. This research, led by Faezeh Saghafian from Tehran University of Medical Sciences, reviewed 27 studies to examine the connection between fruit and vegetable consumption and depression. It found that eating more fruits and vegetables is linked to a lower risk of depression, with every 100 g increase reducing the risk by 3%–5%.

Professor Almudena Sánchez-Villegas
Sánchez-Villegas, A., Verberne, L., De Irala, J., Ruiz-Canela, M., Toledo, E., Serra-Majem, L., & Martinez-Gonzalez, M. A. (2011). Dietary fat intake and the risk of depression: The SUN Project. *PLoS One*, *6*(1), e16268. This research, led by Professor Almudena Sánchez-Villegas from the University of Las Palmas de Gran Canaria, examined 12,059 Spanish university graduates and found that higher intake of trans unsaturated fatty acids (TFA) was linked to an increased risk of depression, showing a clear dose–response effect. In contrast, higher intakes of monounsaturated fatty acids (MUFA) and polyunsaturated fatty acids (PUFA), along with olive oil use, were associated with a lower risk of depression.

Ruo-Gu Xiong
Xiong, R. G., Li, J., Cheng, J., Wu, S. X., Huang, S. Y.,

Zhou, D. D., ... & Feng, Y. (2023). New insights into the protection of dietary components on anxiety, depression, and other mental disorders caused by contaminants and food additives. *Trends in Food Science* **&** *Technology*, *138*, **44-56.** This research, led by Ruo-Gu Xiong from Sun Yat-sen University, found that contaminants like heavy metals and pesticides, as well as food additives, can contribute to mental disorders such as anxiety and depression. On the other hand, dietary components like probiotics, fruits, and vegetables were shown to provide protective effects against these conditions.

Yeonji Yang

Yang, Y., Kim, Y., & Je, Y. (2018). Fish consumption and risk of depression: Epidemiological evidence from prospective studies. *Asia-Pacific Psychiatry*, *10*(4), e12335. This research, led by Yeonji Yang from Kyung Hee University, reviewed 10 cohort studies with 109,764 participants and found a modest link between fish and omega-3 fatty acid intake and a reduced risk of depression. The adjusted relative risk for the highest versus lowest fish consumption was 0.89, while for omega-3 intake, it was 0.87.

Step Five: Movement

Majd Alnawwar

Alnawwar, M. A., Alraddadi, M. I., Algethmi, R. A., Salem, G. A., Salem, M. A., & Alharbi, A. A. (2023). The effect of physical activity on sleep quality and sleep disorder: A systematic review. *Cureus*, *15*(8). This research, led by Majd Alnawwar from King Fahad Hospital, reviewed 23 studies on the relationship between physical activity and sleep, emphasising its positive effects on sleep quality and sleep disorders. By analysing data from sources like PubMed and MEDLINE, the review synthesised evidence showing how exercise impacts sleep outcomes. The findings suggest that promoting physical activity could be an effective strategy for addressing sleep-related issues.

Sammi Chekroud

Chekroud, S. R., Gueorguieva, R., Zheutlin, A. B., Paulus, M., Krumholz, H. M., Krystal, J. H., & Chekroud, A. M. (2018). **Association between physical exercise and mental health in 1·2 million individuals in the USA between 2011 and 2015: A cross-sectional study.** *The Lancet Psychiatry,* *5*(9), 739-746. This research, led by Sammi Chekroud from the University of Oxford, involving 1,237,194 US adults, found that exercise was associated with a 43.2% reduction in days of poor mental health. Team sports, cycling, and aerobic activities were particularly effective, with 45-minute sessions 3–5 times a week providing the greatest benefits.

Dr Daniel Collado-Mateo

Collado-Mateo, D., Lavín-Pérez, A. M., Peñacoba, C., Del Coso, J., Leyton-Román, M., Luque-Casado, A., ... & Amado-Alonso, D. (2021). **Key factors associated with adherence to physical exercise in patients with chronic diseases and older adults: An umbrella review.** *International Journal of Environmental Research and Public Health, 18*(4), 2023. This research, led by Dr Daniel Collado-Mateo from Rey Juan Carlos University, analysed 55 studies to identify key factors influencing adherence to physical exercise in patients with chronic diseases and older adults. The review highlighted 14 crucial factors that consistently emerged, including program characteristics, professional involvement, supervision, technology use, participant assessment, education, enjoyment, daily integration, social support, communication, progress monitoring, self-efficacy, active participation, and goal setting.

Saskia Heijnen

Heijnen, S., Hommel, B., Kibele, A., & Colzato, L. S. (2016). **Neuromodulation of aerobic exercise—A review.** *Frontiers in Psychology, 6,* 1890. This research, led by Saskia Heijnen from Leiden University, examined how aerobic exercise, like running, impacts hormones, amino acids, and neurotransmitters. The review suggests that effective exercise programs should be well-structured, avoid overtraining, and take individual differences into account.

Dr Andreas Heissel

Heissel, A., Heinen, D., Brokmeier, L. L., Skarabis, N., Kangas, M., Vancampfort, D., ... & Schuch, F. (2023). Exercise as medicine for depressive symptoms? A systematic review and meta-analysis with meta-regression. *British Journal of Sports Medicine*, *57*(16), 1049-1057. This research, led by Dr Andreas Heissel from the Faculty of Human Science and Faculty of Health Sciences Brandenburg, included 41 studies with 2,264 participants. It found that exercise significantly reduces depressive symptoms compared to non-active controls, with a large effect size (standardised mean difference = −0.946). Supervised and group aerobic exercises were particularly beneficial.

Dr Erin Hoare

Hoare, E., Stavreski, B., Jennings, G. L., & Kingwell, B. A. (2017). Exploring motivation and barriers to physical activity among active and inactive Australian adults. *Sports*, *5*(3), 47. This research, led by Dr Erin Hoare from the Baker Heart and Diabetes Institute, analysed data from the 2015 National Heart Foundation of Australia Heart Week Survey, involving 894 adults aged 25–54. Among inactive individuals (198), the most common barrier to exercise was a lack of time (50.0%).

Professor Erica Jackson

Jackson, E. M. (2013). Stress relief: The role of exercise in stress management. *ACSM's Health & Fitness Journal*, *17*(3), 14-19. This research, led by Professor Erica Jackson from Delaware State University, found that exercise is an effective tool for managing stress, with all types providing benefits. Programs that align with health guidelines can help individuals cope with stress.

Dr Kent Langston

Langston, P. K., Sun, Y., Ryback, B. A., Mueller, A. L., Spiegelman, B. M., Benoist, C., & Mathis, D. (2023). Regulatory T cells shield muscle mitochondria from interferon-γ–mediated damage to promote the beneficial effects of exercise. *Science Immunology*, *8*(89), eadi5377. This research, led by Dr Kent Langston from Harvard Medical School, found that exercise increases muscle regulatory T cells (Tregs), which help prevent excessive production of interferon-γ and mitochondrial disruptions in mice. The absence of Tregs reduced the performance benefits of exercise, suggesting that exercise naturally boosts Tregs and may offer therapeutic advantages for diseases.

Dr Liliana Laranjo

Laranjo, L., Ding, D., Heleno, B., Kocaballi, B., Quiroz, J. C., Tong, H. L., ... & Bates, D. W. (2021). Do smartphone applications and activity trackers increase physical activity in adults? Systematic review, meta-analysis and metaregression. *British Journal of Sports Medicine*, *55*(8), 422-432. This research, led by Dr Liliana Laranjo from the University of Sydney, reviewed the effectiveness of mobile apps and activity trackers with automated feedback in promoting physical activity. By analysing 35 randomised controlled trials involving 7,454 adults, the review found that these interventions had a small-to-moderate positive effect, equating to an increase of about 1,850 steps per day compared to control groups. Notably, interventions that included text messaging and personalisation were particularly effective.

Gabrielle Lindsay Smith

Lindsay Smith, G., Banting, L., Eime, R., O'Sullivan, G., & Van Uffelen, J. G. (2017). The association between social support and physical activity in older adults: A systematic review. *International Journal of Behavioral Nutrition and Physical Activity*, *14*, 1-21. This research, led by Gabrielle Lindsay Smith from Victoria University, reviewed 27 studies to explore how social support and loneliness impact physical activity in older adults. The findings revealed that support specific to physical activity, especially from family members, is positively linked to leisure-time physical activity. However, general social support, support from friends, and loneliness showed mixed associations with activity levels.

Dr Mingli Liu

Liu, M., Wu, L., & Ming, Q. (2015). How does physical activity intervention improve self-esteem and self-concept in children and adolescents? Evidence from a meta-analysis. *PLoS One*, *10*(8), e0134804. This research, led by Dr Mingli Liu from Hunan University of Science and Technology, analysed 25 randomised controlled trials and 13 non-randomised studies involving 2,991 participants to examine how physical activity interventions affect self-esteem and self-concept. The results indicated significant positive effects on general self-outcomes, self-concept, and self-worth.

Kathleen Mikkelsen

Mikkelsen, K., Stojanovska, L., Polenakovic, M., Bosevski, M., & Apostolopoulos, V. (2017). Exercise and mental health. *Maturitas*, *106*, **48-56.** This research, led by Kathleen Mikkelsen from Victoria University, reviewed literature highlighting the positive effects of exercise on mood states like anxiety, stress, and depression. The benefits were attributed to physiological mechanisms such as endorphin release, neurotransmitter regulation, and reduced inflammation, along with psychological factors like distraction and increased self-efficacy. Exercise was found to lower inflammation through multiple pathways as well.

US National Institute on Aging

National Institute on Aging. (2001). *Exercise: A guide from the National Institute on Aging (No. 1)*. **National Institute on Aging.** This guide from the US National Institute on Aging offers practical advice for older adults on staying active. It covers various types of exercises—endurance, strength, balance, and flexibility—and provides tips for safe and effective workouts. The guide emphasises the health benefits of regular exercise, such as improved mobility, enhanced mental health, and greater independence as people age.

Dr Cristy Phillips

Phillips, C., & Salehi, A. (2016). A special regenerative rehabilitation and genomics letter: Is there a "hope" molecule? *Physical Therapy, 96*(4), 581-583. This research, led by Dr Cristy Phillips from Arkansas State University, explores how regenerative rehabilitation and genomics can enhance treatments for mood disorders like depression. It highlights the importance of "hope molecules", such as PGC-1α, which are released during exercise and may positively affect brain mechanisms related to depression.

Dr Gro Samdal

Samdal, G. B., Eide, G. E., Barth, T., Williams, G., & Meland, E. (2017). Effective behaviour change techniques for physical activity and healthy eating in overweight and obese adults; Systematic review and meta-regression analyses. *International Journal of Behavioral Nutrition and Physical Activity, 14,* 1-14. This research, led by Dr Gro Samdal from the University of Bergen, reviewed 48 randomised controlled trials to evaluate behaviour change techniques (BCTs) for promoting physical activity and healthy eating in overweight and obese adults. The findings highlight that goal setting, self-monitoring, graded tasks, and person-centred approaches like Motivational Interviewing significantly improved short- and long-term outcomes. These techniques were linked to better adherence to healthy habits, emphasising their importance in sustaining lifestyle changes.

Wenjing Yan

Yan, W., Chen, L., Wang, L., Meng, Y., Zhang, T., & Li, H. (2023). Association between enjoyment, physical activity, and physical literacy among college students: A mediation analysis. *Frontiers in Public Health, 11,* 1156160.

This research, led by Wenjing Yan from Beijing Sport University, explored how enjoyment of physical activity (PAE) influences the relationship between moderate to vigorous physical activity (MVPA) and physical literacy (PL) in 1,980 Chinese college students. The results showed that PAE significantly mediates this relationship, accounting for 65.58% of the effect. Both PAE and PL were linked to increased MVPA, emphasising the importance of enjoyment in encouraging physical activity.

Step Six: Social Engagement

Professor Manfred Beutel
Beutel, M. E., Klein, E. M., Brähler, E., Reiner, I., Jünger, C., Michal, M., ... & Tibubos, A. N. (2017). Loneliness in the general population: Prevalence, determinants and relations to mental health. *BMC Psychiatry*, *17*, 1-7. This research, led by Professor Manfred Beutel from Johannes Gutenberg University, analysed data from 15,010 German adults aged 35–74 to explore how loneliness affects health. About 10.5% of participants reported feeling lonely, with loneliness more common in younger adults, women, those without partners, and people living alone. The research linked loneliness to increased risks of depression, anxiety, suicidal thoughts, smoking, and more frequent visits to the doctor.

Dr Daniel Campagne
Campagne, D. M. (2019). Stress and perceived social isolation (loneliness). *Archives of Gerontology and Geriatrics*, *82*, 192-199. This research, led by Dr Daniel Campagne from the Universidad Nacional de Educación a Distancia, examined 42 studies on loneliness, highlighting its connection to biological factors like stress hormones and the immune system. While current treatments focus on the physical and mental effects of loneliness with limited success, the review suggests that addressing the biological aspects directly could provide a new and effective way to manage loneliness.

Centers for Disease Control and Prevention
Centers for Disease Control and Prevention. (2024). Social connectedness. CDC. https://www.cdc.gov/social-connectedness/about/index.html This article from the Centers for Disease Control and Prevention reviews the role of social connectedness and explains how strong social connections can boost both mental and physical health by lowering the risk of depression, anxiety, and chronic diseases. The research shows that social engagement promotes healthier behaviours, like improved eating habits and more physical activity, contributing to overall wellbeing.

Dr Wing-Yee Cheung
Cheung, W. Y., Sedikides, C., & Wildschut, T. (2016).
Induced nostalgia increases optimism (via social-connectedness and self-esteem) among individuals high, but not low, in trait nostalgia. *Personality and Individual Differences*, *90*, 283-288. This research, led by Dr Wing-Yee Cheung from the University of Southampton, explored how nostalgia influences optimism. It found that for people who naturally experience nostalgia, reflecting on the past boosted their optimism by strengthening feelings of social connectedness and self-esteem.

Dr Julianne Holt-Lunstad
Holt-Lunstad, J., Smith, T. B., Baker, M., Harris, T., & Stephenson, D. (2015). Loneliness and social isolation as risk factors for mortality: A meta-analytic review. *Perspectives on Psychological Science*, *10*(2), 227-237. This research, led by Dr Julianne Holt-Lunstad from Brigham Young University, analysed research from 1980 to 2014 to explore how social isolation and loneliness affect early death. It found that being socially isolated, feeling lonely, or living alone increases the risk of dying early by 29%, 26%, and 32%, respectively. These effects were seen in both men and women across different regions, although they varied based on age and initial health.

Dr Julianne Holt-Lunstad
Holt-Lunstad, J., Smith, T. B., & Layton, J. B. (2010).
Social relationships and mortality risk: A meta-analytic
review. *PLoS Medicine, 7*(7), e1000316. This research, led by
Dr Julianne Holt-Lunstad from Brigham Young University,
reviewed 148 studies with over 308,000 participants, finding
that strong social relationships boost the chances of survival by
50%. The positive impact on mortality risk was most
pronounced for those with greater social integration, regardless
of age, gender, or health status.

Dr Elvira Lara
Lara, E., Caballero, F. F., Rico-Uribe, L. A., Olaya, B.,
Haro, J. M., Ayuso-Mateos, J. L., & Miret, M. (2019). Are
loneliness and social isolation associated with cognitive
decline? *International Journal of Geriatric Psychiatry, 34*(11),
1613-1622. This research, led by Dr Elvira Lara from the
Universidad Autónoma de Madrid, followed 1,691 adults aged
50 and older over 3 years, exploring how loneliness and social
isolation affect cognition. It found that loneliness led to poorer
cognitive performance and a quicker decline in cognitive
abilities. Social isolation also had a negative impact on cognitive
function, and these effects remained even after factoring in
depression.

Professor Ming Wen
Lennon, A. (2022, March 22). Social engagement may
improve cognition in pre-dementia. Medical News Today.
https://www.medicalnewstoday.com/articles/social-
engagement-may-improve-cognition-in-pre-dementia
This article provides insights from Professor Ming Wen on
how social engagement can boost cognitive function in people
with pre-dementia. Researchers suggest that staying socially
active helps delay cognitive decline by keeping the brain
stimulated. The concept of "use it or lose it" is emphasised to
maintain cognitive health.

Mengyun Luo

Luo, M., Ding, D., Bauman, A., Negin, J., & Phongsavan, P. (2020). **Social engagement pattern, health behaviours and subjective well-being of older adults: An international perspective using WHO-SAGE survey data.** *BMC Public Health*, *20*, 1-10. This research, led by Mengyun Luo from the University of Sydney, looked at data from 33,338 older adults across 6 low- to middle-income countries as part of the WHO-SAGE study. It found that staying socially engaged is linked to better physical activity and overall wellbeing. However, the influence on smoking, drinking, and diet differed by country. The findings suggest that encouraging social connections can improve health.

Jessica Martino

Martino, J., Pegg, J., & Frates, E. P. (2017). **The connection prescription: Using the power of social interactions and the deep desire for connectedness to empower health and wellness.** *American Journal of Lifestyle Medicine*, *11*(6), 466-475. This research, led by Jessica Martino from Tufts University School of Nutrition, highlights the importance of social connections in lifestyle medicine. It shows that strong social ties can positively influence weight management, blood sugar control, cancer survival, heart disease risk, and mental health. In contrast, social isolation can have detrimental effects. The findings suggest that fostering social connections can enhance both the quality and longevity of life.

Dr Gillian Sandstrom

Sandstrom, G. M., & Dunn, E. W. (2014). **Is efficiency overrated? Minimal social interactions lead to belonging and positive affect.** *Social Psychological and Personality Science*, *5*(4), 437-442. This research, led by Dr Gillian Sandstrom from the University of British Columbia, explored how friendly interactions with service providers, like baristas, can boost happiness. Participants who engaged in social conversations reported feeling more positive compared to those who kept the interactions short. These feelings of increased happiness were linked to a greater sense of belonging.

Dr Stefan Stieger

Stieger, S., Lewetz, D., & Willinger, D. (2023). Face-to-face more important than digital communication for mental health during the pandemic. *Scientific Reports*, *13*(1), 8022. This research, led by Dr Stefan Stieger from Karl Landsteiner University of Health Sciences, involving 411 participants from German-speaking countries, found that face-to-face communication was more important for mental health during the COVID-19 lockdowns than digital communication. While text-based digital interactions (like emails or WhatsApp) had some positive effects, videoconferencing offered minimal benefits. Overall, in-person interactions were significantly more beneficial for mental wellbeing compared to digital communication or physical activities.

Jingyi Wang

Wang, J., Mann, F., Lloyd-Evans, B., Ma, R., & Johnson, S. (2018). Associations between loneliness and perceived social support and outcomes of mental health problems: A systematic review. *BMC Psychiatry*, *18*, 1-16. This research, led by Jingyi Wang from University College London, looked at the impact of loneliness and poor social support on mental health. Covering 34 studies, the review found that people with depression who felt they had low social support experienced worse symptoms and slower recovery. Loneliness also seemed to intensify depression, making recovery more difficult.

World Health Organization

World Health Organization. (2022, March 2). COVID-19 pandemic triggers 25% increase in prevalence of anxiety and depression worldwide. World Health Organization. https://www.who.int/news/item/02-03-2022-covid-19-pandemic-triggers-25-increase-in-prevalence-of-anxiety-and-depression-worldwide This article from the World Health Organization (WHO) reported a 25% increase in global anxiety and depression during the first year of the COVID-19 pandemic. This surge was driven by social isolation, fear, uncertainty, and economic stress. WHO emphasises the need for countries to strengthen mental health services and provide better support for those affected.

Step Seven: Self-Care and Hobbies

Dr Gregory Brown
Brown, G. S. (2022). *The self-healing mind: An essential five-step practice for overcoming anxiety and depression, and revitalizing your life*. Harper Wave. This book, authored by Dr Gregory Brown, offers a 5-step approach to managing anxiety, depression, and mental wellbeing. It combines self-care, mindfulness, spirituality, physical activity, and medication. Dr Brown advocates for holistic mental health practices, encouraging readers to build resilience and take control of their mental wellness for revitalisation.

Dr Lisa Butler
Butler, L. D., Mercer, K. A., McClain-Meeder, K., Horne, D. M., & Dudley, M. (2019). Six domains of self-care: Attending to the whole person. *Journal of Human Behavior in the Social Environment*, 29(1), 107-124. This research, led by Dr Lisa Butler from the University at Buffalo, highlights the importance of self-care for helping professionals to prevent burnout and improve wellbeing. It identifies 6 key areas to focus on—physical, professional, relational, emotional, psychological, and spiritual. The study also provides guidance on creating a personalised self-care plan.

Aimee Daramus
Hsieh, C., & Ali, S. (2024). 116 types of hobbies: Activities and interests to try in 2024. Well+Good. https://www. wellandgood.com/types-of-hobbies/ This article provides insights from Aimee Daramus, listing 116 hobbies across categories like creative arts, food, gaming, indoor/outdoor

activities, and crafting. It highlights how hobbies can boost wellbeing, reduce stress, and promote balance in life. The article encourages exploring various interests to discover activities that bring fulfilment.

Dr Kaylee Crockett
Jones, A. (2023, September 25). Self-care: What is it and why is it so important for your health? University of Alabama at Birmingham News. https://www.uab.edu/ news/youcanuse/item/13176-self-care-what-is-it-why-is-it-so-important-for-your-health This article provides insights from Dr Kaylee Crockett, highlighting the importance of self-care in maintaining overall health. It explains that self-care includes activities that enhance physical, mental, and emotional wellbeing, emphasising that practising self-care regularly is vital for long-term health and resilience.

Dr Elkin Luis
Luis, E., Bermejo-Martins, E., Martinez, M., Sarrionandia, A., Cortes, C., Oliveros, E. Y., ... & Fernández-Berrocal, P. (2021). Relationship between self-care activities, stress and well-being during COVID-19 lockdown: A cross-cultural mediation model. *BMJ Open*, *11*(12), e048469. This research, led by Dr Elkin Luis from the University of Navarra, surveyed 1,082 participants from Chile, Colombia, Ecuador, and Spain during COVID-19 lockdowns. It found that self-care plays a role in reducing the negative effects of stress on psychological wellbeing. The study also highlighted that age influenced this relationship, reinforcing the need to promote self-care and stress management, especially during challenging times.

Dr Alyson Ross
Ross, A., Touchton-Leonard, K., Perez, A., Wehrlen, L., Kazmi, N., & Gibbons, S. (2019). Factors that influence health-promoting self-care in registered nurses: Barriers and facilitators. *Advances in Nursing Science*, *42*(4), 358-373. This research, led by Dr Alyson Ross from the National

Institutes of Health Clinical Center, analysed survey responses to understand what helps or hinders nurses in engaging in health-promoting behaviours. Key barriers included a lack of time, resources, and support, along with fatigue and an unhealthy food culture.

Step Eight: Digital Detox

Daneyal Arshad

Arshad, D., Joyia, U. M., Fatima, S., Khalid, N., Rishi, A. I., Rahim, N. U. A., ... & Salmaan, A. (2021). The adverse impact of excessive smartphone screen-time on sleep quality among young adults: A prospective cohort. *Sleep Science*, *14*(4), 337-341. This research, led by Daneyal Arshad from Rawalpindi Medical University, looked at how smartphone screen time affects sleep quality in 280 medical students over 30 days. Screen time was tracked through an app, while sleep quality was measured using the Pittsburgh Sleep Quality Index. The findings showed that more screen time was linked to worse sleep quality.

Dr Kimberly Burkhart

Burkhart, K., & James R, P. (2009). Amber lenses to block blue light and improve sleep: A randomized trial. *Chronobiology International*, *26*(8), 1602-1612. This research, led by Dr Kimberly Burkhart from the University of Toledo, studied 20 adults who wore either blue-blocking (amber) or yellow-tinted glasses for 3 hours before bed. Although the amber lens group started with poorer sleep quality, after 2 weeks they experienced significant improvements in both sleep quality and mood compared to the control group. The study suggests that wearing amber lenses to block blue light before sleep can boost both sleep and mood.

Digital Health Task Force

Canadian Paediatric Society, Digital Health Task Force. (2017). Screen time and young children: Promoting health

and development in a digital world. *Paediatrics & Child Health*, **22**(8), **461.** This research from the Digital Health Task Force looked at how screen media affects children under 5, covering developmental, psychosocial, and physical health aspects. It emphasises the importance of having evidence-based guidelines for screen use and highlights 4 key principles: minimising screen time, reducing risks, using screens mindfully, and modelling healthy behaviours.

Dr Allana LeBlanc

LeBlanc, A. G., Gunnell, K. E., Prince, S. A., Saunders, T. J., Barnes, J. D., & Chaput, J. P. (2017). The ubiquity of the screen: An overview of the risks and benefits of screen time in our modern world. *Translational Journal of the American College of Sports Medicine*, *2*(17), **104-113.** This research, led by Dr Allana LeBlanc from the University of Ottawa Heart Institute, discusses the development of screen-based sedentary behaviour and its associated risks and benefits. It highlights how too much screen time, although convenient, can negatively affect health. The study reviews historical research and offers evidence on the importance of balancing screen use with physical activity for optimal wellbeing.

Abhinav Mehrotra

Mehrotra, A., Pejovic, V., Vermeulen, J., Hendley, R., & Musolesi, M. (2016, May). My phone and me: Understanding people's receptivity to mobile notifications. In *Proceedings of the 2016 CHI Conference on Human Factors in Computing Systems* **(pp. 1021-1032).** This research, led by Abhinav Mehrotra from the University of Birmingham and University College London, examined how mobile notifications impact response times and perceived disruptions. Involving 20 participants, researchers collected data from over 10,000 notifications and 474 questionnaire responses. The findings revealed that how notifications are presented, the type of alert, and individual user traits all play a significant role in how disruptive notifications feel, even when the content is important.

Sudheer Kumar Muppalla

Muppalla, S. K., Vuppalapati, S., Pulliahgaru, A. R., & Sreenivasulu, H. (2023). Effects of excessive screen time on child development: An updated review and strategies for management. *Cureus, 15*(6). This research, led by Sudheer Kumar Muppalla from the Institute of Medical Sciences and Research, explored how screen time affects children's development by analysing various studies. The systematic review found that, while screens can be beneficial for learning, excessive screen use can harm cognitive, language, and social–emotional development. It also linked high screen time to obesity, sleep disorders, and mental health problems.

Apriana Rahmawati

Rahmawati, A., Muji Fitriana, D., & Pradany, R. N. (2019). A systematic review of excessive social media use: Has it really affected our mental health? *Jurnal Ners, 13*(3). This research, led by Apriana Rahmawati from Universitas Airlangga, examined 15 articles from databases like Scopus, ScienceDirect, and EBSCOhost to investigate the negative effects of excessive social media use on mental health. The findings revealed that spending over 2 hours a day on social media is associated with addiction, particularly among individuals with avoidant attachment styles, who tend to engage with social media in more problematic ways. The review suggests that taking breaks from social media can help reduce perceived stress.

Abida Sultana

Sultana, A., Tasnim, S., Hossain, M. M., Bhattacharya, S., & Purohit, N. (2021). Digital screen time during the COVID-19 pandemic: A public health concern. *F1000Research, 10*, 81. This research, led by Abida Sultana from the Nature Study Society of Bangladesh, discusses how the COVID-19 pandemic led to increased screen time among various groups, potentially harming physical and mental health. It highlights the connection between higher screen time and issues like depression, especially in individuals with sedentary lifestyles.

Yali Zhang
Zhang, Y., Li, S., & Yu, G. (2021). The longitudinal relationship between boredom proneness and mobile phone addiction: Evidence from a cross-lagged model. *Current Psychology, 41*, **1-8.** This research, led by Yali Zhang from Renmin University of China, explored the relationship between boredom proneness and mobile phone addiction in 352 Chinese college students. It found that mobile phone addiction is a stronger predictor of boredom proneness rather than the other way around. This relationship was consistent across genders.

Step Nine: Gratitude

Dr Anna Boggiss
Boggiss, A. L., Consedine, N. S., Brenton-Peters, J. M., Hofman, P. L., & Serlachius, A. S. (2020). A systematic review of gratitude interventions: Effects on physical health and health behaviours. *Journal of Psychosomatic Research, 135*, **110165.** This research, led by Dr Anna Boggiss from the University of Auckland, analysed 19 studies on how gratitude interventions affect physical health and health behaviours. While there were improvements in subjective sleep quality, results for other outcomes, like blood pressure and inflammation, were mixed or not fully explored.

The Mindfulness Awareness Research Center at UCLA
Chowdhury, M. R. (2019). The neuroscience of gratitude and effects on the brain. PositivePsychology.com. https:// positivepsychology.com/neuroscience-of-gratitude/ This article features the Mindfulness Awareness Research Center at UCLA, explaining how gratitude boosts brain function. It

activates areas involved in emotional processing and reward, increasing dopamine and serotonin levels, which lifts mood and improves mental wellbeing. Regular gratitude practices can strengthen happiness pathways in the brain and help lower stress and anxiety.

Dr Robert Emmons
Harvard Health Publishing. (2021). Giving thanks can make you happier. Harvard Health. https://www.health. harvard.edu/healthbeat/giving-thanks-can-make-you-happier This article provides insights from Dr Robert Emmons, a psychology professor at UC Davis, suggesting that gratitude not only improves mental health but also encourages healthier habits. Practising gratitude regularly can boost happiness, strengthen relationships, and increase life satisfaction. It's also shown to lower stress, enhance wellbeing, and even improve physical health by promoting a positive mindset.

Prathik Kini
Kini, P., Wong, J., McInnis, S., Gabana, N., & Brown, J. W. (2016). The effects of gratitude expression on neural activity. *NeuroImage*, *128*, 1-10. This research, led by Prathik Kini from Indiana University, followed 60 participants over 3 months, using fMRI to examine the impact of a gratitude-writing exercise on brain activity. Those who engaged in gratitude writing showed increased brain sensitivity to gratitude in the medial prefrontal cortex and expressed more gratitude in their behaviour compared to the control group, who didn't take part in the writing task.

Dr Alex Korb
Korb, A. (2015). *The upward spiral: Using neuroscience to reverse the course of depression, one small change at a time.* New Harbinger Publications. This book, authored by Dr Alex Korb, explains how small positive changes can help reverse depression by creating an "upward spiral". Drawing on neuroscience, the author offers simple strategies, like practising

gratitude, making decisions, and exercising, which boost brain function and gradually lift mood, breaking the cycle of negativity and supporting long-term mental wellbeing.

Professor Sonja Lyubomirsky
Lyubomirsky, S., & Layous, K. (2013). How do simple positive activities increase well-being? *Current Directions in Psychological Science, 22*(1), 57-62. This research, led by Professor Sonja Lyubomirsky from the University of California, reviewed how positive activities, like expressing gratitude or practising kindness, affect happiness. It looked at factors like how often the activities are done, variety, personal motivation, and how well they fit the individual. The positive-activity model highlights 4 key factors—positive emotions, thoughts, behaviours, and need satisfaction—that influence the impact on wellbeing.

Martin Seligman
Seligman, M. E., Steen, T. A., Park, N., & Peterson, C. (2005). Positive psychology progress: Empirical validation of interventions. *American Psychologist, 60*(5), 410. This research, led by Martin Seligman from the University of Pennsylvania, highlights the growth of positive psychology, focusing on strengths, virtues, and happiness. A study with 6 groups, using random assignment and a placebo-controlled design, tested 5 happiness interventions. Three of these successfully boosted happiness and reduced depression, offering a helpful addition to traditional wellbeing methods.

Shawn Achor
Stillman, J. (2016). The amazing way gratitude rewires your brain for happiness. Inc Australia. https://www.inc. com/jessica-stillman/the-amazing-way-gratitude-rewires-your-brain-for-happiness.html This article features insights from Shawn Achor, explaining how practising gratitude can rewire the brain for greater happiness. It describes how expressing gratitude activates neural pathways linked to joy and positivity, and over time, this can lead to lasting improvements

in mood, resilience, and overall wellbeing, creating a "happiness loop".

Professor Philip Watkins

Watkins, P. C., & McCurrach, D. (2016). Progress in the science of gratitude. In C.R. Snyder et al. (eds.), *Oxford Handbook of Positive Psychology* (3rd ed., pp. 571–585). Oxford Academic. This chapter, from lead author Professor Philip Watkins based out of Eastern Washington University, reviews recent developments in gratitude research, including its key benefits and challenges. It covers 4 types of gratitude interventions: recounting, reflection, expression, and reappraisal. The authors argue that gratitude boosts wellbeing by enhancing positive thinking, relationships, and self-perception.

Professor Murat Yıldırım

Yıldırım, M., & Alanazi, Z. S. (2018). Gratitude and life satisfaction: Mediating role of perceived stress. *International Journal of Psychological Studies, 10*(3), 21-28. This research, led by Professor Murat Yıldırım from the University of Leicester, involving 141 Arabic-speaking undergraduate students, used self-report questionnaires to measure gratitude, life satisfaction, and stress. The results showed that gratitude was linked to higher life satisfaction, while stress was linked to lower satisfaction. Mediation analysis found that stress fully mediated the relationship, meaning higher gratitude improved life satisfaction by reducing stress.

Dr Hongbo Yu

Yu, H., Gao, X., Zhou, Y., & Zhou, X. (2018). Decomposing gratitude: Representation and integration of cognitive antecedents of gratitude in the brain. *Journal of Neuroscience, 38*(21), 4886-4898. This research, led by Dr Hongbo Yu from Peking University, involved 24 participants and used fMRI during a social interaction task to explore how the brain processes gratitude. It found that the perigenual anterior cingulate cortex integrates the benefactor's cost and the recipient's benefit, creating a sense of gratitude. The study also linked gratitude to reciprocal behaviour through specific brain connections.

Step Ten: Cognitive Behaviour Therapy

Dr Judith Beck

Beck, J. S. (2020). *Cognitive behavior therapy: Basics and beyond*. **Guilford Publications.** This book, authored by Dr Judith Beck, presents key techniques supported by detailed case studies and practical tips. It includes new chapters on therapeutic relationships and mindfulness, introducing recovery-oriented cognitive therapy. Enhanced with clinical tips, practice exercises, and videos, the book also incorporates strategies from Acceptance and Commitment Therapy, Dialectical Behaviour Therapy, and other therapeutic approaches.

Dr Stefan Hofmann

Hofmann, S. G., Asnaani, A., Vonk, I. J., Sawyer, A. T., & Fang, A. (2012). The efficacy of cognitive behavioral therapy: A review of meta-analyses. *Cognitive Therapy and Research*, *36*, 427-440. This research, led by Dr Stefan Hofmann from Boston University, analysed 106 out of 269 meta-analyses on cognitive behaviour therapy (CBT) for various issues, including anxiety, depression, and psychotic disorders. The findings strongly support CBT for anxiety disorders, somatoform disorders, bulimia, anger, and stress, often showing it to be more effective than other treatments.

Professor Steven Hollon

Hollon, S. D., DeRubeis, R. J., Andrews, P. W., & Thomson Jr, J. A. (2021). Cognitive therapy in the treatment and prevention of depression: A fifty-year retrospective with an evolutionary coda. *Cognitive Therapy and Research*, *45*(3), 402-417. This research, led by Professor Steven Hollon from Vanderbilt University, examines the effectiveness of cognitive therapy compared to antidepressants for nonpsychotic depression, referencing various studies and neural imaging data. The analysis shows that cognitive therapy lowers relapse rates by improving cortical regulation of emotions, while medications typically dampen stress responses. It suggests that cognitive therapy may be more effective than medication alone in promoting problem-solving and emotional regulation.

Avy Joseph

Joseph, A., & Chapman, M. (2013). *Confidence and success with CBT: Small steps to achieve your big goals with cognitive behaviour therapy.* **John Wiley & Sons.** This book, authored by Avy Joseph, provides practical CBT techniques for boosting confidence and motivation, and overcoming anxiety and low self-esteem. It serves as a comprehensive guide for addressing and changing negative thought patterns and behaviours, making it a valuable resource for individuals and therapists seeking to enhance their personal and professional lives.

S.J. Scott and Barrie Davenport

Scott, S. J., & Davenport, B. (2016). *Declutter your mind: How to stop worrying, relieve anxiety, and eliminate negative thinking.* **Oldtown Publishing.** This book, authored by S.J. Scott and Barrie Davenport, offers practical strategies to reduce overthinking, manage anxiety, and enhance mental clarity. It emphasises mindfulness, prioritising tasks, and eliminating negative thought patterns to boost emotional wellbeing. The book encourages readers to create mental space for positivity and focus on what truly matters in life.

Julie Tseng

Tseng, J., & Poppenk, J. (2020). Brain meta-state transitions demarcate thoughts across task contexts exposing the mental noise of trait neuroticism. *Nature Communications, 11*(1), 1-12. This research, led by Julie Tseng from Queen's University, presents methods for detecting neural meta-state transitions without needing prior data. These transitions align with narrative events, predict new thoughts, and correlate with brain regions associated with spontaneous thinking. The study offers a new way to observe resting cognition and supports mental noise theory by linking transition rates to trait neuroticism.

Lawrence Wallace

Wallace, L. (2017). *Cognitive behavioral therapy: 7 ways to freedom from anxiety, depression, and intrusive thoughts.* **Independently published.** This book, authored by Lawrence Wallace, provides practical CBT techniques to manage and overcome negative thought patterns. It outlines 7 strategies to break free from anxiety and depression, promoting mental clarity and emotional balance by reframing thoughts and altering behaviour patterns.

Dr Jesse Wright

Wright, J. H., Brown, G. K., Thase, M. E., & Basco, M. R. (2017). *Learning cognitive-behavior therapy: An illustrated guide* **(2nd ed.). American Psychiatric Association Publishing.** This book, led by author Dr Jesse Wright, from the University of Louisville, combines 23 new videos with comprehensive text, charts, and tools to effectively teach CBT to non-professional users. It covers core theories, session structuring, and therapeutic relationships, with updates on suicide risk, integration of related therapies, and additional resources for improved learning and practice.

Complementary Approaches

Dr Gaétan Chevalier

Chevalier, G., Sinatra, S. T., Oschman, J. L., Sokal, K., & Sokal, P. (2012). Earthing: Health implications of reconnecting the human body to the earth's surface electrons. *Journal of Environmental and Public Health*, *2012*(1), 291541. This research, led by Dr Gaétan Chevalier from the University of California at Irvine, explores the health benefits of earthing (or grounding), which involves direct physical contact with the Earth's electrons, like walking barefoot or using conductive systems. It highlights emerging research indicating that our modern disconnection from this natural contact may contribute to various health issues. Reconnecting with the Earth's electrons has been linked to improved sleep and reduced pain, suggesting significant clinical potential for this simple and accessible practice.

Julia Doets

Doets, J. J., Topper, M., & Nugter, A. M. (2021). A systematic review and meta-analysis of the effect of whole body cryotherapy on mental health problems. *Complementary Therapies in Medicine, 63,* **102783.** This research, led by Julia Doets from the Mental Health Service Organization, reviewed 10 studies on whole-body cryotherapy for mental health issues, including 6 randomised controlled trials with 294 participants. It found a large overall effect size for mental health improvements (Hedges' $g = 1.63$) and a very large effect specifically for depressive symptoms (Hedges' $g = 2.95$).

Didrik Espeland

Espeland, D., de Weerd, L., & Mercer, J. B. (2022). Health effects of voluntary exposure to cold water–A continuing subject of debate. *International Journal of Circumpolar Health, 81*(1), **2111789.** This research, led by Didrik Espeland from the Arctic University of Norway, systematically analysed 104 studies on cold water immersion (CWI) and its health effects. It found that CWI can significantly influence various physiological and biochemical parameters, including reducing body fat, improving insulin sensitivity, and potentially providing protection against cardiovascular and metabolic diseases.

Dr Robert Golden

Golden, R. N., Gaynes, B. N., Ekstrom, R. D., Hamer, R. M., Jacobsen, F. M., Suppes, T., ... & Nemeroff, C. B.

(2005). The efficacy of light therapy in the treatment of mood disorders: A review and meta-analysis of the evidence. *American Journal of Psychiatry*, *162*(4), 656-662. This research, led by Dr Robert Golden from the University of North Carolina, assessed the effectiveness of light therapy for mood disorders by systematically analysing 8 randomised controlled trials from PubMed. Meta-analyses indicated that bright light treatment and dawn simulation were effective for both seasonal affective disorder and non-seasonal depression, with effect sizes comparable to those of antidepressant medications.

Dr Margaret Hansen

Hansen, M. M., Jones, R., & Tocchini, K. (2017). Shinrin-yoku (forest bathing) and nature therapy: A state-of-the-art review. *International Journal of Environmental Research and Public Health*, *14*(8), 851. This research, led by Dr Margaret Hansen from the University of San Francisco, systematically examined 64 studies on Shinrin-yoku (forest bathing) published between 2007 and 2017. It explored the physiological and psychological benefits of nature exposure, particularly focusing on research from Japan and China. The review suggests that Shinrin-yoku could be an effective method for reducing stress and burnout.

Dr Joy Hussain

Hussain, J., & Cohen, M. (2018). Clinical effects of regular dry sauna bathing: A systematic review. *Evidence-Based Complementary and Alternative Medicine*, *2018*(1), 1857413. This research, led by Dr Joy Hussain from RMIT University, systematically reviewed 40 clinical studies, including 13 randomised controlled trials, to evaluate the health effects of regular dry sauna bathing. Most studies suggest potential benefits, including reducing stress, improving mood, alleviating symptoms of depression and anxiety, and enhancing overall relaxation.

Dr Wesam Kooti

Kooti, W., & Daraei, N. (2017). A review of the antioxidant activity of celery (Apium graveolens L). *Journal of Evidence Based Complementary & Alternative Medicine, 22*(4), 1029-1034. This research, led by Dr Wesam Kooti from Kurdistan University of Medical Sciences, included 9 studies examining the antioxidant activity of celery (Apium graveolens L). It found that celery contains compounds like caffeic acid and luteolin, which have strong antioxidant properties. The review highlights celery's ability to neutralise free radicals.

Dr Jari Laukkanen

Laukkanen, T., Laukkanen, J. A., & Kunutsor, S. K. (2018). Cardiovascular and other health benefits of sauna bathing: A review of the evidence. *Mayo Clinic Proceedings, 93*(8), 1111-1121. This research, led by Dr Jari Laukkanen from the University of Eastern Finland, summarises the epidemiological, experimental, and interventional evidence on the health benefits of Finnish sauna bathing. It includes data from observational studies, randomised controlled trials, and non-randomised controlled trials. The review found that sauna bathing is associated with an 80% reduced risk of developing neurocognitive diseases, along with significant reductions in the risk of cardiovascular and other health conditions.

Dr Christopher Moyer

Moyer, C. A., Rounds, J., & Hannum, J. W. (2004). A meta-analysis of massage therapy research. *Psychological Bulletin, 130*(1), 3-18. This research, led by Dr Christopher Moyer from the University of Illinois Urbana-Champaign, reviewed 37 studies using random assignment to evaluate the effectiveness of massage therapy (MT). It found that single MT sessions reduced state anxiety, blood pressure, and heart rate. Multiple sessions were effective in reducing delayed pain, with the most significant effects on trait anxiety and depression. The benefits of MT were comparable to those of psychotherapy.

Dr Shigeo Ohta

Ohta, S. (2015). Molecular hydrogen as a novel antioxidant: Overview of the advantages of hydrogen for medical applications. *Methods in Enzymology,* **555, 289-317.** This research, led by Dr Shigeo Ohta from the Nippon Medical School, re-evaluates the role of molecular hydrogen (H_2) in mammalian cells, demonstrating its ability to neutralise harmful oxidants like hydroxyl radicals and peroxynitrite. H_2 was shown to be safe and beneficial, with potential applications in preventing and treating various diseases. Administration methods include inhalation and drinking H_2-water. The paper highlights H_2's anti-inflammatory, antiallergic, and antiapoptotic properties, along with its potential for clinical use due to its effectiveness and minimal adverse effects.

Dr Nikolai Shevchuk

Shevchuk, N. A. (2008). Adapted cold shower as a potential treatment for depression. *Medical Hypotheses,* **70(5), 995-1001.** This research, led by Dr Nikolai Shevchuk from the Virginia Commonwealth University School of Medicine, explored the hypothesis that depression may arise from the absence of evolutionary stressors like brief temperature changes and genetic predispositions. It suggested cold showers (20 °C for 2–3 minutes) as a potential treatment, based on evidence that cold exposure activates the sympathetic nervous system and can alleviate depressive symptoms.

Dr Ami Sperber

Sperber, A. D., Bangdiwala, S. I., Drossman, D. A., Ghoshal, U. C., Simren, M., Tack, J., ... & Palsson, O. S. (2021). Worldwide prevalence and burden of functional gastrointestinal disorders, results of Rome Foundation Global Study. *Gastroenterology,* **160(1), 99-114.** This research, led by Dr Ami Sperber from Ben-Gurion University, investigated the prevalence and factors associated with 22 functional gastrointestinal disorders (FGIDs) across 33 countries. Data from 73,076 adults revealed that 40.3% of online respondents met the criteria for at least one FGID, with a higher prevalence in women. FGIDs negatively affected quality of life and led to increased healthcare visits.

Natasha Williams

Williams, N., & Weir, T. L. (2024). Spore-based probiotic Bacillus subtilis: Current applications in humans and future perspectives. *Fermentation*, *10*(2), 78. This research, led by Natasha Williams from Colorado State University, examined human intervention studies on Bacillus subtilis as a probiotic, focusing on its effects on gastrointestinal health. It discusses the stability and effectiveness of B. subtilis spores, their impact on gut microbiota, and related health biomarkers. The paper summarises findings on various strains and explores future applications of B. subtilis in human health.

Dr Shuduo Zhou

Zhou, S., Su, M., Shen, P., Yang, Z., Chai, P., Sun, S., ... & Chen, K. (2024). Association between drinking water quality and mental health and the modifying role of diet: A prospective cohort study. *BMC Medicine*, *22*(1), 1-12. This research, led by Dr Shuduo Zhou from Peking University, included 24,285 participants from the Yinzhou Cohort (2016–2021) and investigated the relationship between metal and nonmetal elements in drinking water and depression and anxiety. The study found that manganese reduced the risk of depression, while copper and cadmium increased it. Additionally, anxiety risk rose with exposure to manganese, iron, and selenium.

Glossary

Amygdala: The amygdala is a small, almond-shaped part of the brain that plays a key role in processing emotions, especially fear, stress, and anxiety. It helps us respond to threats or stressful situations by triggering "fight or flight" reactions. The amygdala also helps store emotional memories, so we can learn from past experiences.

Antioxidants: Antioxidants are substances that help protect our cells from damage caused by unstable molecules called free radicals. Think of them as tiny defenders that keep our bodies healthy and protect against ageing and diseases.

Biopsychosocial model: The biopsychosocial model is a way of understanding health by looking at the whole picture. It considers not just the physical aspects but also psychological factors and social influences that can affect a person's wellbeing.

Brain plasticity: Brain plasticity, or neuroplasticity, is the brain's ability to change and adapt throughout life. It means the brain can reorganise itself by forming new connections, helping us learn new skills and recover from injuries.

Cortisol: Cortisol is a hormone produced by the adrenal glands that helps regulate stress, metabolism, and the immune system. It's often called the "stress hormone" because its levels rise in response to stress and help our body cope.

Dopamine: Dopamine is a chemical in the brain that helps control movement, motivation, and pleasure. It's often called the "feel-good" neurotransmitter because it plays a key role in how we experience enjoyment and reward.

Gut–brain axis: The gut–brain axis is the connection between our digestive system and our brain. It's a communication network where signals travel back and forth, affecting everything from mood to digestion and overall mental health.

Inflammation: Inflammation is our body's natural response to injury or infection. It's like a protective reaction where our immune system sends extra blood and cells to the affected area. While it helps with healing, chronic inflammation can lead to health problems.

Meta-analysis: A meta-analysis combines results from multiple studies on the same topic to find overall trends and conclusions. It uses statistical methods to pool data and provide a more precise estimate of effects or relationships.

MTHFR gene: The *MTHFR* gene provides instructions for making an enzyme involved in processing folate (vitamin B9) and regulating homocysteine levels. Variations in this gene can affect how well you metabolise these substances, which can impact health.

Neurotransmitters: Neurotransmitters are chemical messengers in the brain that help transmit signals between nerve cells. They play a key role in mood, sleep, focus, and many other functions by carrying information across the nervous system.

Norepinephrine: Norepinephrine is a neurotransmitter and hormone that helps control your body's fight-or-flight response. It boosts alertness, focus, and energy, and also helps regulate mood and stress levels.

Oxidative stress: Oxidative stress is when there are too many unstable molecules in our bodies, which can damage our cells. It's like having too much rust in a machine—if not controlled, it can lead to health problems.

Placebo: A placebo is a treatment or substance with no active ingredients, such as a sugar pill or dummy procedure, used in experiments to see if a real treatment works better than just believing we're being treated. It can also sometimes make people feel better just because they think they're getting help.

Serotonin: Serotonin is a chemical in the brain that helps regulate mood, sleep, and appetite. Often called the "feel-good" neurotransmitter, it helps us feel happy and balanced.

Systematic review: A systematic review is a thorough and organised way of looking at all the research on a specific topic. Researchers collect, evaluate, and summarise existing studies to give a clear picture of what's known and what needs more investigation.

Wellbeing: Wellbeing is a broad term that refers to overall health and happiness. It includes feeling good physically, mentally, and emotionally, and having a sense of satisfaction and balance in our life.